Partnerships for Mental Health

Laura Weiss Roberts • Daryn Reicherter
Steven Adelsheim • Shashank V. Joshi

Editors

Partnerships
for Mental Health

Narratives of Community
and Academic Collaboration

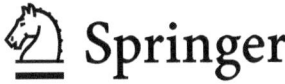 Springer

Editors
Laura Weiss Roberts, MD, MA
Department of Psychiatry
   and Behavioral Sciences
Stanford University School of Medicine
Stanford, CA, USA

Steven Adelsheim, MD
Department of Psychiatry
   and Behavioral Sciences
Stanford University School of Medicine
Stanford, CA, USA

Daryn Reicherter, MD
Department of Psychiatry
   and Behavioral Sciences
Stanford University School of Medicine
Stanford, CA, USA

Shashank V. Joshi, MD
Department of Psychiatry
   and Behavioral Sciences
Stanford University School of Medicine
Stanford, CA, USA

ISBN 978-3-319-18883-6   ISBN 978-3-319-18884-3   (eBook)
DOI 10.1007/978-3-319-18884-3

Library of Congress Control Number: 2015946564

Springer Cham Heidelberg New York Dordrecht London

Printed on acid-free paper

Springer International Publishing AG Switzerland is part of Springer Science+Business Media (www.springer.com)

To Eric and our family

—Laura

To Amelia, Ethan, and Heidi: you are the wind in my sails and you inspire me to try to make the world a better place for all.

—Daryn

To my wife, Tara, whom I met in a community collaborative meeting. Through both your work and personal interactions, you continue to daily teach me the true meaning of community partnership.

—Steve

To the schools in the San Francisco Bay Area that we have been privileged to walk alongside of and grow with. A special thanks to Malathy, Aanand, Amrit, and Sanjan for their loving support and for tolerating the many late-night arrivals after community meetings.

—Shashank

Foreword

Partnerships Between Academic Medical Centers and Community-Based Organizations Enhance the Mission and Impact of Each

To address the complexity of modern challenges and opportunities, partnerships are increasingly important in a variety of different disciplines. This book presents meaningful and moving examples of partnerships between members of academic medical centers (AMCs) (e.g., faculty, students, and staff) and community-based organizations (e.g., clients, patients, leaders, volunteers, and workers). The examples described in these chapters provide tangible evidence of the positive impact that these partnerships have had, and continue to have, on the health and welfare of individuals and communities.

I am particularly pleased and grateful that many of the community partnerships described in this book have been developed by Stanford faculty. I also appreciate the role of Dr. Laura Weiss Roberts, Chairman of the Department of Psychiatry and Behavioral Sciences at Stanford University School of Medicine, and her departmental colleagues, Drs. Daryn Reicherter, Steven Adelsheim, and Shashank Joshi, in encouraging these partnerships and in editing this book.

AMCs have had a critically important role in virtually all major biomedical advances over the past century. The groundbreaking report of Abraham Flexner in 1910 [1] identified the need for a scientifically based curriculum in medical schools. The implementation of recommendations from the Flexner report led to the formation of AMCs with tripartite and interrelated missions of patient care, research, and teaching. Diagnosis and treatment of diseases were advanced, innovations abounded, and patient care improved—particularly for patients with acute illnesses who were treated within the four walls of a hospital. Communities have certainly benefitted from the Flexner revolution, but only more recently have AMCs viewed outreach to communities and partnerships with community-based organizations as an integral part of their broad mission to improve human health.

As we look to the future, community partnerships, such as those described in this book, will be of increasing importance to the core mission of AMCs, which is evolving to focus on a broader view of health as something more than just medical care for acute illnesses. This mission is evolving for at least three reasons. First, many scientific opportunities compel us to look at the mission of an AMC as being broader than the diagnosis and treatment of disease. We now have within our grasp the opportunity to make major advances in the prediction and prevention of disease, thereby adding a new dimension to the scope of engagement and impact of AMCs. Second, integrated and coordinated approaches over long periods of time are required to provide effective care for patients with multiple medical problems. This need compels us to broaden our scope of focus to include effective care for patients with chronic diseases in addition to our traditional focus on acute diseases. Third, as expressed in a number of ways, society now expects all of us involved in the delivery of health care in America to be much more focused on value (e.g., improved outcomes at lower cost).

Community partnerships will be essential for success in each of these areas. Collaboration with community partners is needed to promote well-being and stop disease before it starts—from providing local screenings to ensuring vaccine compliance. As more and more individuals cope with chronic disease, community initiatives increasingly provide programs that support healthy habits, like smoking cessation and exercise—areas often forgotten in the provision of medical care. Finally, as we work toward improving value in health care, greater coordination across medical and social and community service providers will play a key role in sustaining long-term health in a cost-effective manner.

Another factor that is pushing AMCs toward increasing community partnerships is an increased awareness of the social determinants of health—the conditions in which we are born, live, and work—and the prominent and yet often unacknowledged role these conditions play in our well-being. Abraham Flexner himself recognized the importance of social factors, asserting that physicians have the duty "to promote social conditions that conduce to physical well-being" [1, p. 68]. The function of a physician, he noted more than a century ago, "is fast becoming social and preventive, rather than individual and curative" [1, p. 26].

The programs and activities described in each of the chapters of this book provide compelling examples of passionate commitment, unfailing optimism, and steadfast persistence. We learn about Lawrence McGlynn's personal journey as a boy growing up in the San Francisco Bay Area during the early years of the HIV epidemic [2]. McGlynn's perspectives evolve during his transitions to medical school, residency in psychiatry, and appointment as a faculty member. His desire to improve the lives of those with HIV and methamphetamine addiction and to bring the epidemic into check led him to provide care to patients at the Partners in AIDS Care and Education (PACE) Clinic in San Jose and the Positive Care Clinic at Stanford. In addition to the care he provides as a psychiatrist, McGlynn has been involved in educating health care workers and community members about the linkage between methamphetamine addiction and HIV. His work has also included studies and interventions aimed at reducing methamphetamine use.

Suzanne Walker and Victor Carrion [3] describe the effects of chronic stress and trauma on the health of children and youth in a San Francisco community. A dose–response relationship has been demonstrated between adverse childhood experiences (including physical neglect and abuse, emotional neglect and abuse, sexual abuse, and substance abuse in the household) and adult risk of chronic disease. Walker, Carrion, and their colleagues developed the Center for Youth Wellness with collocated pediatric medical and mental health services as a part of a federally qualified heath center in Bayview Hunters Point (a residential neighborhood of San Francisco that has experienced high rates of poverty, community violence, and adverse environmental exposure). They found that 12 % of the children in this community were affected by four or more adverse childhood experiences, and 51 % of these children were identified as having learning and behavioral problems. Evidence-based therapies have been developed through partnerships that include teachers, pediatricians, psychiatrists, dentists, and nutritionists.

On the international front, the chapter of the book written by Jayne Fleming and Daryn Reicherter [4] describes how a group of physicians and human rights lawyers came together to send a legal-medical delegation to Haiti a month after the devastating magnitude 7.0 earthquake in 2010. Reicherter, a psychiatrist and recognized expert in cross-cultural trauma, led the medical team. Fleming, a pro bono attorney at Reed Smith LLP, led the legal team. They and their colleagues went to Haiti to understand the human rights situation and to identify individuals who might qualify for evacuation due to extraordinary circumstances, such as medical conditions that could not be treated in Haiti. Thirty-seven candidates for humanitarian parole were identified during their first visit, all of whom were victims of rape and suffered from posttraumatic stress disorder.

This first visit to Haiti led to an enduring commitment, and volunteers with the Haiti Humanitarian Project have since made about 30 more trips to the country, working closely not only with community groups but also with the United Nations High Commissioner for Refugees. When faced with financial and logistical challenges on the ground, the team has persevered and developed innovative solutions. They have used cutting-edge telehealth technology to help assess whether or not people met criteria for refugee status. By late 2014, the group had succeeded in permanently resettling 52 Haitian women and children in the United States and Canada.

The partnerships described in this book provide an exciting glimpse into the transformative effects of partnerships between communities and the faculty, students, and staff at AMCs. I have focused on three of the narratives, but each story provides unique understanding of how collaboration can bring about positive change.

Such improvement is urgently needed, as there remains much room for improvement on the health care landscape. The United States has some of the best hospitals in the world, and American patients have earlier access to cutting-edge drugs and treatments and generally shorter waiting times to see physicians. But on broad measures of health outcomes like infant mortality and life expectancy, the United States ranks near the bottom among the countries belonging to the Organization for Economic Coordination and Development. Moreover, improvement on these types of indicators is slower in the United States than in most other nations.

AMCs have an important role in addressing these shortcomings. To realize our potential, we need to expand our mission beyond *care* to include *health*—and not just for individuals but also for communities. By partnering with community-based organizations, AMCs are increasingly focusing on prevention, chronic disease, health care value, the social determinants of health, and other significant factors that contribute to human health and well-being on a broad scale.

We live in a time of enormous potential for biomedical discovery and improvements in human health. Collaboration between community and academic partners will play a critically important role in realizing this potential. The collaborations highlighted in this book are inspired examples of what can be accomplished.

Lloyd B. Minor, M.D.

References

1. Flexner A. Medical education in the United States and Canada: A report to the Carnegie Foundation for the Advancement of Teaching. New York: The Carnegie Foundation for the Advancement of Teaching; 1910.
2. McGlynn LM. The Stanford–Santa Clara County Methamphetamine Task Force. In: Roberts LW, Reicherter D, Adelsheim S, Joshi S, editors. Partnerships for mental health: narratives of community and academic collaboration. New York: Springer Science+Business Media, LLC; 2015.
3. Walker SE, Carrion VG. The Center for Youth Wellness: A community-based approach to holistic health care in San Francisco. In: Roberts LW, Reicherter D, Adelsheim S, Joshi S, editors. Partnerships for mental health: narratives of community and academic collaboration. New York: Springer Science+Business Media, LLC; 2015.
4. Fleming JE, Reicherter D. The earthquake. In: Roberts LW, Reicherter D, Adelsheim S, Joshi S, editors. Partnerships for mental health: narratives of community and academic collaboration. New York: Springer Science+Business Media, LLC; 2015.

Preface

I lived in New Mexico 10 years before I wore a western-style belt, so deep was my intention to not appear other than what I was—a kid from Chicago who loved the sky, the mountains, the high desert, and the green chile of New Mexico.

I trained and worked at the medical school, and each year I marveled at the young physicians who would come and, within days of their arrival, don tall cowboy hats and boots, denim of a particular cut, and silver and turquoise. These men and women would come for adventure, enticed by what was novel to them in this large, sparsely and diversely populated frontier. These young healers came to New Mexico promising to learn and to dedicate their efforts to a place rich with poverty, need, and risk. Some of these young physicians stayed (usually trading their initial Southwest costume for a more subtle bolo tie or earrings). And yet, many of these same men and women would leave. They were unhappy with all that was unfamiliar to them. They were exhausted by the demands of a rural, relentlessly resource-poor place. Commitments made to individuals and to the communities of New Mexico no longer held, and, the sense of promise was no longer felt.

A second, more positive observation from this formative time in the Southwest relates to the ingenuity that arises in situations of overwhelming need and few resources. A great example is a program developed decades ago by a child psychiatrist from the university who was working in a frontier community in which many adolescent girls were becoming pregnant and dropping out of school. These young mothers and their children were experiencing tremendous mental and physical health challenges. Most were not doing well at all. Their futures were becoming diminished and the entire community was affected. Efforts by teachers and local leaders to "educate" young people about birth control and pregnancy over many years were essentially ineffective. Working with the community, the psychiatrist came up with an idea: to develop a toddler care program and, in this carefully supervised setting, to employ young teenage girls as the caregivers. Through one initiative, many of the older adolescent mothers in the community were able to return to school, bringing far more salutary outcomes to their families. But another effect was felt among the adolescent girls working in the toddler program: seeing how difficult it was to take care of little kids, the teenagers made considerable efforts to avoid becoming pregnant. The pattern was disrupted.

Another great example of necessity as the "mother of invention" was a collaboration over nearly two decades that has brought together state, county, and university partners to address the overwhelming needs of elders who reside in remote areas throughout New Mexico and have serious mental illnesses, such as depression, anxiety, late-life psychosis, and dementia. Few resources exist for this greatly burdened special population of New Mexico. New Mexico is the fifth-largest state in the United States, with 0.6 % of the country's population, so most of the state qualifies as truly frontier (i.e., fewer than 6 people per square mile), and it has few clinics, hospitals, and health professionals. New Mexico also is economically distressed, currently ranked 48 out of 50 states with respect to fiscal health, with one in five individuals living below the poverty line. And New Mexico, like other rural states, has an overrepresentation of children, elders, and disabled individuals. Alone, the state could never do enough. The counties could never do enough. The university could never do enough. Together, however, the three partners could bring different elements from which an effective program could be, and was, built. The state contributed resources, novel solutions for reimbursing home-based care, and networking with a broader system; the counties contributed local clinic and generalist clinician efforts; and the university contributed subspecialty expertise, clinical trainees, continuing education, and respite support. In this program, a circuit-riding faculty physician traveled the state—working side-by-side with community-based colleagues, performing clinic, home, and video visits with rural elders and their families, and training physicians interested in rural health care.

My work in academic-community partnering has evolved since my early days in New Mexico and, even before, in urban underserved communities of Chicago. I have had the privilege in my academic work to engage with individuals from all walks of life and most places throughout the world. In my work at Stanford Medicine, we now have activities and initiatives in our neighborhood and across the globe. Several of the stories of these partnerships are told in this book. Other partnership narratives shared here are those of my friends, and of the friends of my friends.

Partnerships for Mental Health: Narratives of Community and Academic Collaboration is a text that follows from an earlier work that Christiane Brems, Ph.D., Mark Johnson, Ph.D., and I created with many remarkable colleagues. That book, *Community-Based Participatory Research for Improved Mental Healthcare: A Manual for Clinicians and Researchers*, was published in 2013 (also by Springer Science+Business Media). The manual laid the foundation for this collection, which has a greater focus on partnerships as experienced by those who create them.

This next book richly tells the stories of collaboration. The narrative voice of each chapter derives from the people who tell their story. Authors of this book are immigrants, survivors of torture, mental health experts, urban people, rural people, teachers, doctors, attorneys, students, and international leaders. Their stories matter. These authors provide emotionally powerful tales that will, I believe, move, affect, and encourage those who encounter them in this book. Stories are influential. This collection of narratives is inspired by these individuals, who believe that collaboration can bring authentic mutualism, promise-keeping, and innovation to address the hardest problems we face as a world community.

Stanford, CA, USA   Laura Weiss Roberts, M.D., M.A.

Acknowledgements

The editors wish to thank their many colleagues who generously shared their experiences and insights for the book.

We express our appreciation to Melina Salvador, who helped in the early developmental stages of this project, and to Madcline McDonald Lane-McKinley, Ph.D.(cand.), Jennifer Pearlstein, and Megan Cid for their assistance at various stages in the preparation of the book.

The editors and authors wish to express their utmost gratitude to Ann Tennier for her dedication, hard work, and attention to detail on this book project. Her contribution was appreciated throughout the development of the project and can be seen throughout the finished product.

The editors and authors also wish to thank Diane Lamsback and Richard Lansing of Springer Science+Business Media, LLC.

Contents

Contributors

Steven Adelsheim, M.D. Department of Psychiatry and Behavioral Sciences, Stanford University School of Medicine, Stanford, CA, USA

Paula Alvarez, Ph.D. Pacific Graduate School of Psychology, Palo Alto University, Palo Alto, CA, USA

Rania Awaad, M.D. Department of Psychiatry and Behavioral Sciences, Stanford University School of Medicine, Stanford, CA, USA

Michele Barry, M.D. Stanford University School of Medicine, Stanford, CA, USA

John Battaglia, M.D. Department of Psychiatry, University of Wisconsin School of Medicine and Public Health, Madison, WI, USA

Sophany Bay, M.H.R.S Gardner Family Care Corporation, Cambodian Program, San Jose, CA, USA

James K. Boehnlein, M.D., M.Sc. Department of Psychiatry, Oregon Health and Science University, Portland, OR, USA

Caroline Bonham, M.D., M.S. Department of Psychiatry and Behavioral Sciences, University of New Mexico Health Sciences Center, Albuquerque, NM, USA

Kurt Buske, M.S.W. Consultant

Veronica Cardenas, Ph.D. Department of Psychiatry, University of California, San Diego, San Diego, CA, USA

Victor G. Carrion, M.D. Department of Psychiatry and Behavioral Sciences, Stanford University School of Medicine and Lucile Packard Children's Hospital, Stanford, CA, USA

Margaret Cary, M.D., M.P.H. Division of Child and Adolescent Psychiatry, Department of Psychiatry, Oregon Health and Science University, Portland, OR, USA

Tith Chan, M.H.T., A.S.W. Gardner Family Care Corporation, Cambodian Program, San Jose, CA, USA

Keith Cheng, M.D. Division of Child and Adolescent Psychiatry, Department of Psychiatry, Oregon Health and Science University, Portland, OR, USA

Gloria J. Coleman, B.A., M.S. Institute of Juvenile Research, Chicago, IL, USA

Geri R. Donenberg, Ph.D. School of Public Health and College of Medicine, University of Illinois at Chicago, Chicago, IL, USA

Jack Drescher, M.D. New York Medical College, New York, NY, USA; William A. White Institute, New York, NY, USA; New York University, New York, NY, USA

Paul Dunlap, M.F.A., M.S. English Department, Henry M. Gunn Senior High School, Palo Alto, CA, USA

Jayne E. Fleming, J.D. Firm Reed Smith LLP, New York, NY, USA

Brenikki R. Floyd, Ph.D., M.P.H. Community Outreach Intervention Projects, School of Public Health, University of Illinois at Chicago, Chicago, IL, USA

Chris Fore, Ph.D. Department of Behavioral Health, IHS TeleBehavioral Health Center of Excellence, Albuquerque, NM, USA

Dolores Gallagher-Thompson, Ph.D., A.B.P.P. Department of Psychiatry and Behavioral Sciences, Stanford University School of Medicine, Stanford, CA, USA

Joe Glass, M.S. Department of Behavioral Health, Mescalero Indian Hospital, Mescalero, NM, USA

Cheryl Gore-Felton, Ph.D. The Office of Academic Affairs, Stanford University School of Medicine, Stanford, CA, USA; Department of Psychiatry and Behavioral Sciences, Stanford University School of Medicine, Stanford, CA, USA

Samantha N. Hartley, B.A. Department of Psychiatry and Behavioral Sciences, Stanford university School of Medicine, Stanford, Palo Alto, CA, USA

Hannah Holt, M.S. Department of Clinical Psychology, Palo Alto University, Palo Alto, CA, USA

Keith Humphreys, Ph.D. Center for Innovation to Implementation, Veterans Affairs and Stanford University Medical Centers, Menlo Park, CA, USA

Roya Ijadi-Maghsoodi, M.D. Health Services Research and Development Center, VA Greater Los Angeles Healthcare System, Los Angeles, CA, USA

Shaili Jain, M.D. Department of Psychiatry and Behavioral Sciences, Stanford University School of Medicine, Stanford, CA, USA; VA Palo Alto Health Care System, Menlo Park, CA, USA

Kaela Joseph, M.S. VA Palo Alto Health Care System, Menlo Park, CA, USA

Shashank V. Joshi, M.D. Department of Psychiatry and Behavioral Sciences, Stanford University School of Medicine, Stanford, CA, USA

Sheryl Kataoka, M.D., M.S.H.S. Division of Child and Adolescent Psychiatry, UCLA Semel Institute, Los Angeles, CA, USA

Christina Tara Khan, M.D., Ph.D. Department of Psychiatry and Behavioral Sciences, Stanford University School of Medicine and Veterans Affairs Palo Alto Health Care System, Stanford, CA, USA

J. David Kinzie, M.D., F.A.C.Psych. Department of Psychiatry, Oregon Health and Science University, Portland, OR, USA

Cheryl Koopman, Ph.D. Department of Psychiatry and Behavioral Sciences, Stanford University School of Medicine, Stanford, CA, USA

Joseph B. Layde, M.D., J.D. Department of Psychiatry and Behavioral Medicine, Medical College of Wisconsin, Milwaukee, WI, USA

Yeon Soo Lee, M.H.T, L.C.S.W Gardner Family Care Corporation, APYP/Cambodian Program, San Jose, CA, USA

Paul K. Leung, M.D. Department of Psychiatry, Oregon Health and Science University, Portland, OR, USA

Steven E. Lindley, M.D., Ph.D. Department of Psychiatry and Behavioral Sciences, Stanford University School of Medicine, Stanford, CA, USA; VA Palo Alto Health Care System, Menlo Park, CA, USA

Lawrence McGlynn, M.S., M.D. Department of Psychiatry and Behavioral Sciences, Stanford University School of Medicine, Stanford, CA, USA

Yvonne Aida Maldonado, M.D. Department of Pediatrics, Stanford University, Stanford, CA, USA

Sarah Estes Merrell, M.A. St. Ignatius College Preparatory, San Francisco, CA, USA

Lloyd B. Minor, M.D. Carl and Elizabeth Naumann Dean of the Stanford University School of Medicine, Stanford, CA, USA

Bophal Phen, M.H.T., L.C.S.W Gardner Family Care Corporation, Cambodian Program, San Jose, CA, USA

Claudia L. Reardon, M.D. Department of Psychiatry, University of Wisconsin School of Medicine and Public Health, Madison, WI, USA

Daryn Reicherter, M.D. Department of Psychiatry and Behavioral Sciences, Stanford University School of Medicine, Stanford, CA, USA

Laura Weiss Roberts, M.D., M.A. Department of Psychiatry and Behavioral Sciences, Stanford University School of Medicine, Stanford, CA, USA

Craig S. Rosen, Ph.D. National Center for PTSD Dissemination and Training Division, Menlo Park, CA, USA; VA Palo Alto Health Care System, Menlo Park, CA, USA; Department of Psychiatry and Behavioral Sciences, Stanford University School of Medicine, Stanford, CA, USA

David Wyatt Seal, Ph.D. Tulane University School of Public Health and Tropical Medicine, Global Community Health and Behavioral Sciences, New Orleans, LA, USA

Behjat Sedighi, Q.M.H.P. Department of Psychiatry, Oregon Health and Science University, Portland, OR, USA

Dorlynn Simmons, M.S.S.W. Mescalero Service Unit, Mescalero, NM, USA

Leonard Thomas, M.D. Indian Health Service, Albuquerque Area Office, Albuquerque, NM, USA

Lorie Van Tilburg, M.S.W. Southern Caregiver Resource Center, San Diego, CA, USA

Marian Tzuang, M.S.W. Stanford University School of Medicine, Stanford Geriatric Education Center, Stanford, CA, USA

Roberto E. Velasquez, M.S. Southern Caregiver Resource Center, San Diego, CA, USA

Art Walaszek, M.D. Department of Psychiatry, University of Wisconsin School of Medicine and Public Health, Madison, WI, USA

Suzanne E. Walker, M.A. San Francisco State University, San Francisco, CA, USA

Helen W. Wilson, Ph.D. Department of Psychiatry and Behavioral Sciences, Stanford University School of Medicine, Stanford, CA, USA

About the Editors

Laura Weiss Roberts, M.D., M.A., serves as Chairman and the Katharine Dexter McCormick and Stanley McCormick Memorial Professor in the Department of Psychiatry and Behavioral Sciences at the Stanford University School of Medicine. She is an internationally recognized scholar in bioethics, psychiatry, medicine, and medical education. Dr. Roberts has received many honors as well as extensive scientific peer-reviewed funding from the National Institutes of Health, the Department of Energy, and private foundations to perform empirical studies of modern ethical issues in research, clinical care, and health policy, with a particular focus on vulnerable and special populations. Her work has led to advances in understanding of ethical aspects of physical and mental illness research, societal implications for genetic innovation, the role of stigma in health disparities, the impact of medical student and physician health issues, and optimal approaches to fostering professionalism in medicine. Dr. Roberts owns Terra Nova Learning Systems.

Steven Adelsheim, M.D., serves as Clinical Professor and Director of Community Partnerships in the Department of Psychiatry and Behavioral Sciences in the School of Medicine at Stanford University. He is also Professor Emeritus at the University of New Mexico Health Sciences Center. Dr. Adelsheim has partnered in developing mental health policy and systems, including those focused on school mental health, telebehavioral health, tribal programs, and suicide prevention at local, regional, state, and national levels. Dr. Adelsheim has also focused on creating and implementing early detection/intervention programs for young people in school-based and primary care settings, including programs for those with depression, anxiety, and prodromal/early psychosis symptoms. Over the years, he has received primary funding from the Robert Wood Johnson Foundation, the Substance Abuse and Mental Health Services Administration, and the National Institute of Mental Health.

Daryn Reicherter, M.D., serves as Clinical Associate Professor in the Department of Psychiatry and Behavioral Sciences in the School of Medicine at Stanford

University. His work centers on cross-cultural trauma mental health. He has been involved in the creation of clinical mental health programs for underserved populations in the San Francisco Bay Area. He is an attending psychiatrist at the Center for Survivors of Torture, Asian Americans for Community Involvement. He works with refugee survivors from around the world. Dr. Reicherter is involved with the movement for promotion of trauma mental health and human rights issues spanning countries including Cambodia, Haiti, Zimbabwe, and Indonesia. He has ongoing involvement in advocacy for human rights through the Human Rights in Trauma Mental Health Laboratory, an interdisciplinary group of academic faculty advocating for the use of mental health outcomes in international human rights criminal and immigration law. He has published articles, chapters, and books on the topic of cross-cultural trauma. He serves as consultant to the Documentation Center of Cambodia for the Victims of Torture Project.

Shashank V. Joshi, M.D., serves as an Associate Professor and Director of Training in Child and Adolescent Psychiatry in the Department of Psychiatry and Behavioral Sciences at Stanford University. He has a faculty appointment in the Department of Pediatrics and in the School of Education at Stanford University, and he leads school-based mental health services in partnership with Lucile Packard Children's Hospital. Dr. Joshi is the recipient of numerous awards in teaching and public service, including a Mental Health Provider Hero Award in Suicide Prevention from the County of Santa Clara, California. Dr. Joshi's academic focus is on the effectiveness of school mental health and therapeutic interventions in pediatric health. He has published and lectured widely on therapist-family-teacher collaboration in medical care, cultural aspects of pediatric health, and suicide prevention in school settings.

Introduction

The giant pine tree grows from a tiny seedling.
A tower nine stories high starts with a single brick.
A journey of a thousand miles begins with a single step.

Lao Tzu

If you want to walk fast, walk alone.
If you want to walk far, walk together.

Russian proverb

Beginning with a Single Step

Mental disorders represent the second-leading cause of disease burden in the world. Only infectious diseases surpass neuropsychiatric, addiction, and related conditions in human suffering, as measured by years of life lost due to early death and severe disability. Affected are people living in cities, in rural areas, in economically established countries, and in economically emerging countries. Affected are people of all ages, both genders, in minority and ethnically distinct communities, in majority communities, and in all strata of society. In seeking to lessen the burden of mental disorders, the obstacles are many: insufficient resources, insufficient expertise, insufficient infrastructure. And then there is stigma. Stigma is pervasive—worsening the suffering experienced by individuals with mental disorders, heightening the barriers in seeking care, and interfering with the creation of adequate systems of care.

Addressing mental health concerns throughout the world is truly a very hard problem. Very hard problems of this nature matter a great deal, and they require innovation and collaboration to resolve. This book is about the stories of innovation and collaboration occurring between community and academic partners who have undertaken among the very hardest of problems—the care of veterans with ravaging posttraumatic stress disorder; the care of homeless individuals with HIV, addiction, and mental illness; the care of caregivers for Hispanic family members with Alzheimer's disease; the prevention of illness in impoverished vulnerable youth; and the rescue of profoundly mentally ill earthquake survivors. This book also tells the story of identity formation of early-career physicians with a calling to work with distinct populations for whom suffering and stigma are immense. This book also tells the stories of the special bonds that develop and are strengthened between community members and academic colleagues and, ultimately, between friends.

With these narratives, we invite the reader to see how partnerships emerge around a specific, very hard problem and how efforts toward a solution unfold. These narratives offer perspectives on partnerships, documenting the process of working together, reflecting the creativity and fellowship of collaboration, and displaying the different architectures of effective community-academic partnerships. Partnerships between community-based and academic collaborators are intended to bring value in the present, bringing resources and services to make a difference in real time. Reflecting on the process and results of partnerships clarify which approaches may be replicated or adapted to help others elsewhere, making a difference in the future.

Our aim in developing this collection is thus to illustrate and inspire collaboration in order to bring about better health outcomes for people affected by mental health issues in communities throughout the world. Each journey has its beginning. We invite you to join with us in taking the single step of this book's journey.

Laura Weiss Roberts, M.D., M.A.
Daryn Reicherter, M.D.
Steven Adelsheim, M.D.
Shashank V. Joshi, M.D.

Narrative 1
The Stanford–Santa Clara County Methamphetamine Task Force

Lawrence McGlynn

This is a story of an academic physician collaborating with social workers, other health professionals, and local organizers to establish solutions for a community highly affected by HIV/AIDS and methamphetamine abuse.

Central Moment

I have made the walk from the Civic Center BART station to Davies Symphony Hall dozens of times, winding my way through four blocks of the homeless and hungry. One evening in 2004 as I hurried along the familiar trek, a skeleton of a man wearing an unbuttoned shirt, swimming in threadbare khakis, and engaged in an angry conversation with himself was briskly walking on a head-on collision course towards me. Ten feet of distance granted me recognition of this man's face. His empty eyes and sunken cheeks could not distort my memory. Two feet of distance provided him recognition of my face. His self-dialogue ceased and he ran away. I knew this man as a patient who had sat in my office on countless occasions, but 3 months earlier he had vanished. A graduate degree in engineering did not prevent him from becoming HIV-positive nor shield him from methamphetamine. That evening I sat in the symphony while he was running in the Tenderloin, a neighborhood of drugs, guns, and violence. That same evening I appreciated how the strings

L. McGlynn, M.S., M.D. (✉)
Department of Psychiatry and Behavioral Sciences,
Stanford University School of Medicine, Stanford, CA, USA
e-mail: lmcglynn@stanford.edu

© Springer International Publishing Switzerland 2015
L.W. Roberts et al. (eds.), *Partnerships for Mental Health*,
DOI 10.1007/978-3-319-18884-3_1

needed the woodwinds, the percussions needed the brass, and together, beautiful music was created. I had to let go of the idea that I could fix this on my own. This man and those like him needed a full orchestra.

Introduction

In *Madness and Civilization*, Foucault described the role leprosy played in European society. Lepers, recognized as ones to be feared, were an excluded class and existed both physically and culturally on the outer edges of the "healthy" community.

> At the end of the Middle Ages, leprosy disappeared from the Western world. In the margins of the community, at the gates of cities, there stretched wastelands which sickness had ceased to haunt but had left sterile and long uninhabitable [1].

Human Immunodeficiency Virus (HIV) and Acquired Immune Deficiency Syndrome (AIDS), not unlike leprosy, has had a physical and a cultural presence. Community-based groups founded early in the epidemic, most notably ACT UP,[1] expressed concerns that those living with HIV were being viewed as second-class citizens, ostensibly ignored by the government in the 1980s and avoided by the society at large. The groups encouraged challenging the status quo and sought to empower the afflicted, many of whom were themselves members of these organizations.

Today the treatment of HIV/AIDS has allowed those with the virus to feel optimistic about the future. They are living longer, returning to work, and having children. The optimism is appropriate, as the HIV viral load[2] can be controlled with medications. Absolute CD4+ T cell counts[3] in many cases can be brought into the normal range. Difficulties, however, still remain. Stigma continues in many communities and has been identified as a risk factor for depression [2]. Cognitive impairment, fatigue, and sexual dysfunction are common complaints. Some patients with these symptoms have learned to look outside allopathic medicine for relief. Eastern medicine has been used in HIV since the beginning of the epidemic, when there were no medications available, and has included acupuncture and herbal remedies. Other treatments, however, may or may not safely ameliorate patients' health. Methamphetamine use, which temporarily increases energy, concentration, mood, and sexual function, has become a path to feeling better for some HIV-positive individuals. Unfortunately it is not without significant physical, mental, or public health risks. Academic and community groups have recognized these consequences and have come together in many of the affected regions to address this barrier to the health of those living with and without HIV. The Stanford–Santa Clara County Methamphetamine Task Force adopted the mission of reducing methamphetamine use in the San Francisco Bay Area, with a particular emphasis on those living with, or at risk of acquiring, HIV.

---

[1] ACT UP, the AIDS Coalition to Unleash Power, formed in New York in 1987, in part, to make available treatment for those living with HIV/AIDS.

[2] The number of HIV RNA copies per milliliter of blood plasma, and an important parameter of immune function.

[3] As HIV disease progresses without medications, this count will characteristically drop, leaving the individual vulnerable to opportunistic infections.

How Did I Get Here?

The memories of aromatic eucalyptus trees growing in the hills of Dominican invite me to think more deeply about childhood, leading me back to wonderful recollections, but once again deceiving me and re-inciting the pain. I remember cardboard slides and lizards. I remember nuns walking in pairs on warm summer evenings. I remember picking pomegranates from our neighbor's tree. I remember the Westminster Quarters lofting out of St. Raphael's campanile, the bells subsequently chiming a designated number of times to specify the hour on the clock.

But I also remember when the ringing was accompanied by visions of stars and feelings of dizziness, nausea, and shame. I knew it was not the church bells. A simple melody could not possibly activate so many regions of my then 12-year-old brain. More than likely it was a rock, a ball, or a fist with which someone had once again bashed me in the head. Rare was the witness who would protest the attacks, or even help me up. I would clumsily rise on my own, dissociated from the laughing spectators. Those beautiful Marin County children, abundant in numbers and impeccably dressed in parochial school uniforms, were able to fire stinging barbs with amazing accuracy. The events would replay themselves in waves of anticipation on Sunday nights and oftentimes felt more painful than when they actually occurred. Children in my position would consider suicide. Others would turn to drugs for pain relief, and sex for validation. Some would become sick and die before they turned 20.

The Virus

I struggle to say with certainty when I first became aware of the existence of HIV. Life was becoming good for me, as I was now riding on a trajectory from the bullying in Marin to newfound acceptance in San Francisco. Some new force, however, was spoiling the celebration. Young, otherwise healthy gay men in the San Francisco Bay Area were falling ill. The ones who were not bedridden might be seen walking tenuously with canes, perhaps also attempting to cover up the reddish-brown plaques of Kaposi's sarcoma.[4] Rummage sales would spontaneously appear on any sidewalk in the Castro,[5] the sad faces of the vendors reluctantly parting with boxes of well-worn Levis, leather jackets, and flashy disco albums. Local reports of

---

[4] Kaposi's sarcoma is a tumor caused by the human herpes virus 8, and one of the AIDS-defining illnesses.

[5] The Castro is a neighborhood in San Francisco with a large number of LGBT residents and businesses.

"gay cancer" would become national news. In 1982, Tom Brokaw and Robert Bazell offered one of the first network news reports on AIDS:

> Scientists at the National Centers for Disease Control in Atlanta today released the results of a study, which shows that the lifestyle of some male homosexuals has triggered an epidemic of a rare form of cancer [3].

With that report and the deaths of so many San Franciscans, I appreciated the power of the word *cue*. Those events reignited my fear that the world was not a safe place, especially for a person like me. A growing suspicion of gay people, seen by some as a community of disease and culpability, was the sentiment that had now infected the mainstream. My cue was the bell ringing in my head telling me to run and hide in the safety of academia and begin a new chapter in my life. Was I leaving behind a sinking ship full of friends and fellow San Franciscans crying for help? This feeling was the burden I would carry with me into medical school.

> Carlos and Carmen Vidal just had a child
> A lovely girl with a crooked smile
> Now they gotta split 'cause the Bronx ain't fit
> For a kid to grow up in
> Let's find a place they say, somewhere far away
> With no Blacks, no Jews and no Gays
> There but for the grace of God go I [4]

Welcome to Harvard

Anatomy at Harvard Medical School was a gift. We were four students per cadaver being led by Professor Farish Jenkins, who, before each lecture, would use colored chalk to create detailed polychromatic drawings rivaling the artwork of Frank Netter.[6] The laboratory was full of beautiful people who willed themselves to advance medicine. Bodies with HIV, however, were not acceptable. We would see the tarred lungs of smokers and the girth of the morbidly obese, but we would not see the coalesced lesions of PML[7] in a person who died from AIDS.[8]

A series of experiences during my clinical years would sublimate my lingering sense of guilt into choices reflective of my profound desire to help those living and dying with HIV. Seeing patients with Jerome Groopman[9] at the Deaconess; studying

---

[6]Frank H. Netter (1906–1991) was an American surgeon widely known for his medical illustrations.

[7]PML stands for progressive multifocal leukoencephalopathy, a disease of the white matter of the brain, seen almost exclusively in those who are immunocompromised.

[8]Medical schools may not accept an anatomical gift for a variety of reasons, including autopsy, embalming, emaciation, obesity, advanced decomposition, and a history of contagious disease, including HIV/AIDS.

[9]Dr. Groopman has been a staff writer for *The New Yorker* since 1998 and is Chair of Medicine at Harvard Medical School, Boston, MA.

suicide in HIV/AIDS with Alexandra Beckett[10] at the Beth Israel; watching the expertise and sensitivity of Marshall Forstein[11] as he utilized the razor-sharp virtual scalpel of a psychiatrist to enter the subcortex of a 46-year-old transgendered woman with AIDS—these were the experiences that would erase any doubts I had about where I belonged in the field of medicine.

New York City

Fifteen years after the report on *NBC Nightly News* [3], I was a first-year internal medicine resident at St. Vincent's Medical Center in New York's Greenwich Village, arguably the heart of the HIV epidemic. The hospital was one of the first to address and treat HIV and AIDS in the 1980s and was featured in Tony Kushner's play *Angels in America*. By 1986, one third of the hospital's beds were filled with those with AIDS [5]. Some of those who would survive into the next year received high doses of zidovudine, the first antiretroviral medication approved for HIV, AIDS, and ARC.[12] By the time I stepped into the hospital in 1996, many of those with HIV/AIDS continued to require hospitalization. Central nervous system involvement was common in these patients. Performing lumbar punctures would become a routine procedure for most of us interns.

The work was physically and emotionally exhausting. Thankfully the majority of my attending physicians at St. Vincent's were compassionate, patient, and sensitive men and women. Others were not. As if possessing divining rods, those clinicians recognized my weaknesses and pimped[13] them out of me. At times I felt hatred and anger towards those doctors, but in the same minute I was grateful to them for working with the people I cherished so much. I learned a lot that year, but perhaps the toughest lesson was accepting the reality that even health care providers could harbor bigotry. I always looked forward to seeing one particularly smiley and cherubic MICU[14] nurse with a Jamaican accent. One evening I overheard her referring to a patient struggling to stay alive as "another faggot with AIDS." Her voice suddenly sounded like a mis-tuned violin bringing cacophony to an otherwise flawless performance. Fighting the battle with her did not seem to be a choice available to me at that moment. As an intern, I was keenly aware that a nurse could make my life wonderful or miserable, or so I told myself. In truth, fear overtook my judgment and I regret it deeply. To this day I mentally fight the battle with that nurse when I am stuck in traffic, when I have insomnia, and when I have nothing better to do. Perhaps even in the symphony I am hypervigilant for the one instrument or performer who misses a note and reduces the hues of my thoughts from countless grays to the immaturity of black and white.

---

[10] Dr. Beckett is an HIV psychiatrist at Beth Israel Deaconess Medical Center and Harvard Medical School, Boston, MA.

[11] Dr. Forstein is an HIV psychiatrist at Cambridge Hospital Campus of Cambridge Health Alliance and Harvard Medical School, Boston, MA.

[12] ARC is AIDS-related complex.

[13] The meaning of the verb form of *pimp* includes the practice of asking a student questions for the purpose of testing his or her knowledge and is otherwise referred to as the Socratic method.

[14] An MICU is a medical intensive care unit.

Back to Harvard

For an internist, time with patients can seem too brief. Looking to my future in HIV/ AIDS, I wanted to continue training as an internist, but I also recognized its limitations. My longing for more time—just a little more time—was a feeling that also resonated among my dying patients and their families. I made the decision to return to Harvard and enter the psychiatric residency training program at The Cambridge Hospital.[15] With this opportunity I was able to continue learning internal medicine but had the gift of more time with patients as I focused on the complexities of the central nervous system and human behavior. It was the perfect fit. In my final year of training I served as chief resident of the Zinberg Clinic, The Cambridge Hospital's multidisciplinary HIV unit. Team huddles at Zinberg were ahead of their time and offered the opportunity for collaboration between staff, providers, and community members. Huddles also gave us the necessary time to garner moral and emotional support from colleagues, as many patients with AIDS were continuing to die in heartbreaking numbers in the late 1990s. I finished residency in 2000 and accepted an academic-clinical position at Stanford University after being away from the West Coast for 8 years. This opportunity came with a huge amount of happiness about returning home, but also the irrational fear that I would find a postapocalyptic San Francisco consisting of deserted streets, dead gardens, fading Victorians, and the realization that I was too late.

Welcome to Stanford

As I transitioned from residency to my first position as a new attending physician at Stanford, I was to split my time between San Jose, California, and Stanford. Partners in AIDS Care and Education, otherwise known as the Ira Greene PACE Clinic, is a Stanford training site located in San Jose and serves as the largest public health medical facility in Santa Clara County dedicated to those living with HIV/AIDS. It is a community clinic staffed with physicians, therapists, social workers, a nutritionist, a pharmacist, nurses, and a team of benefits counselors. Many of the patients are uninsured or underinsured, over 50 % of whom are Hispanic. Most of the staff members speak Spanish and several speak Vietnamese, both languages commonly heard in the clinic and the surrounding community.

I found my office in the PACE Clinic to be ideal, blessed with a tall but narrow window facing the Santa Cruz mountains. I was scheduled to work at the PACE Clinic on Mondays, Wednesdays, and Fridays. On my first day the clinic manager brought me a catalog of acceptable office art and sterile institutional furniture. My notion of becoming ensconced in a wood-paneled space with a couch, swivel chair,

---

[15] The Cambridge Hospital is now referred to as the Cambridge Hospital Campus of Cambridge Health Alliance.

and oil paintings of Dutch peasants and hunting dogs was not to be realized. Instead, I opted for a large leatherette La-Z-Boy knockoff and two Diego Rivera posters in frosted metal frames. I could not have been happier. The first poster, *Baile en Tehuantepec* ("Dance in Tehuantepec"), shows the working class of Mexico happily dancing, drenched in a sea of bright colors. The second poster, *Cargador de flores* ("The Flower Carrier"), portrays a woman standing above a kneeling man, hands reaching towards him as he is attempting to carry a large bushel of flowers. Would I be the woman helping my patient carry his burden, or the man inviting my patient to pile her troubles on my back? Maybe my roles would change.

On Tuesdays and Thursdays I would spend my days at Stanford in the Positive Care Clinic, a smaller facility serving insured HIV-positive patients and located in a one-story bungalow across from the Stanford Hospital. My practice at both clinics filled up quickly, but within a matter of months the demand for appointments was slowing down. Why was my quiet, distant yet reflective approach not working? Some accused me of being judgmental in my silence. This interpretation could not have been further from the truth. Behind my icy façade, I was cheering these survivors and crying for their losses. I wanted to tell them I loved them and thank them for not giving up. I wanted to tell them that they reminded me of people I knew long ago. My positive countertransference was raging, but so was their negative transference. I learned that I had to be real and soften my boundaries. Silence became dialogue. Handshakes became hugs. Nods became laughter. I used as much tissue as the patients. Business turned around and my biggest challenge has been ending my sessions on time.

$$p = mv$$

Momentum is the product of mass and velocity. How does one calculate the mass of suffering? How can one measure the velocity of an epidemic that began decades earlier and continued to take lives? This linear, conserved quantity carried the dying from the 1980s and 1990s to the 2000s. Although the life-saving cocktail of medications was now becoming more widely available, the momentum had already been established and was too powerful for many of the war weary to successfully battle.

I had seen death as a medical student and as a resident, and it was never easy. But now I was a Stanford attending physician and these were my patients. There was the young man rejected by his family who would come in, close his eyes, and sleep for his allotted half hour. I convinced myself that this treatment was therapeutic, even if only to serve as a chance for him to escape from his reality. Perhaps it was therapeutic for me too. I would not take my eyes off of him, sharing his peace, and quietly hoping he would never die. Within 5 months he lost the battle. There was the woman with four children, at most five teeth in her mouth, and an unforgettable beauty and sweetness to her face that the deep creases could not hide. Her addiction to methamphetamine gave her enough energy and paranoia to distract her from the painful knowledge that the system now had custody of her children. She lived for 2 years after I met her. And then there was the young man who had lymphoma in his brain and a devoted mother by his side. Over the course of 6 months he would gradually lose his ability to recognize me. Our relationship went from office visits to home visits, and culminated with my delivering the eulogy at his funeral. Memorials and services were the norm, and each brought with it a new set of loved ones trying to say goodbye too soon to the sensitive young man or brave young woman they had just lost. For some attendees, however, closure was beyond their reach. Within each church, hall, or synagogue one would notice that lone person sitting in the back corner, shoulders hunched with angst, and head bowed heavily with regret, never again having the opportunity to apologize for rejecting the deceased.

Tina

As the momentum was slowing in 2003, evidenced in part by fewer obituaries in the *Bay Area Reporter*,[16] the medical community would deservedly celebrate the research accomplished and the antiretroviral cocktails now available. Many patients did not need to see their primary care providers every week or month, for now they could get back to their lives and decrease the frequency of their laboratory and clinic visits. My practice, however, became even busier. People who had been living with impending death for so many years now needed to face their own sense of guilt, loss, and symptoms of posttraumatic stress. These feelings, at times referred to as the Lazarus Syndrome, have been likened to the suffering of Holocaust survivors, people who watched their families and friends die and fully expected to follow, but instead were at once freed to a changed and lonely world [6]. A new picture was emerging, one which would begin to define the next chapter of my life at Stanford. The life-saving medications were reducing the number of cases of dementia, but the prevalence of the milder forms of cognitive dysfunction was increasing. Some were also suffering from lipodystrophy,[17] leaving the affected feeling demoralized and exposed. Hypogonadism was not uncommon among the male patients, characterized by sexual dysfunction and depressed mood. Medications such as exogenous testosterone could help some with this condition. Many, however, were turning to "dealers" for relief. Patients found a treatment that gave them energy, increased their libido, improved their attention and concentration, and allowed them to feel pleasure, even if for a limited period of time. This choice, however, did not come without a cost.

During the period of 2003–2005, the use of methamphetamine was becoming more obvious at the PACE Clinic and, to a lesser extent, at the Positive Care Clinic. The drug was relatively inexpensive; however, many would obtain their supply in

---

[16] The *Bay Area Reporter* is a weekly newspaper in San Francisco, California, for the LGBT community. The obituary section would recount the lives of many of those who died from AIDS or AIDS-related causes.

[17] Lipodystrophy is a disfiguring condition characterized by lipoatrophy of the face and limbs and lipohypertrophy of the abdomen and dorsocervical region and is caused in part by certain older antiretroviral medications.

exchange for sex. For others, 20 dollars was the price for a "bag" containing approximately four "hits," enough to keep some people high for several days. Our patients would present themselves to the clinic desperately wanting to sleep or escape the psychosis. Weight loss and poor dentition were not uncommon. A large number had lost their homes, jobs, and relationships, and many were facing criminal charges for drug possession or theft. I was amazed that these patients would show up for their appointments at all. Still, it was almost impossible to predict the demeanor and appearance of the methamphetamine-intoxicated patient. Some patients seemed calm and focused. The "tweaker" stereotype, however, accurately described many who were using the drug chronically. I would see psychomotor agitation as I attempted to make sense of their pressured speech, much of which was nothing more than verbal responses to internal stimuli. Their paranoid delusions were complex dramas involving the FBI, hidden cameras, spying neighbors, and perhaps their nosey psychiatrist secretly monitoring their behavior. Some had delusional parasitosis, convinced that their bodies were covered in bugs. Open sores on their faces and arms were common and evidence to them that the "bugs" were eating their flesh. The PACE Clinic has a small room with a microscope that the infectious disease doctors use to examine specimens. This microscope was now being used more frequently to look at the pieces of lint or clothing fibers that the patients believed were parasitic creatures devouring their skin.

Some patients would stop taking their HIV medications when they were on a "run."[18] Others would continue to take their medications but would also take other drugs, including gamma hydroxybutyrate ("GHB" or "G"), ketamine ("K"), marijuana, benzodiazepines, and MDMA (3,4-methylenedioxy-N-methylamphetamine, also known as "ecstasy," "E," or "X"). Because methamphetamine can cause erectile dysfunction, patients would also use phosphodiesterase type 5 inhibitors (including sildenafil, tadalafil, and vardenafil) and amyl (or butyl) nitrate ("poppers"), the combination of which can be lethal.

"Party and play" (PNP) was frequently the venue in which people, MSM[19] in particular, would use methamphetamine. A typical PNP meeting would include two or more men using methamphetamine (and likely other drugs) and having sex. Because methamphetamine affects judgment, patients were presenting with evidence of engaging in unprotected sex, including higher rates of syphilis, gonorrhea, chlamydia, and Hepatitis C. New HIV infections were increasingly due to PNP methamphetamine use. In fact, almost one in three MSM who tested HIV-positive in 2004 said they had used crystal methamphetamine, representing nearly triple the rate of those MSM who had tested positive for HIV in 2001 [7]. As researchers were learning more about methamphetamine, the picture became increasingly alarming. Literature was confirming what we were learning from our patients: the drug not

---

[18] A "run" is a period of time, generally multiple consecutive days, in which the individual will use methamphetamine without abstinence.

[19] MSM refers to men who have sex with men.

only stimulated arousal but also decreased sexual inhibition and led to the seeking of multiple sex partners and riskier sexual practices, including unprotected intercourse [8]. Those who did become infected with HIV were at an increased risk of depression and fatigue [9], symptoms that may have led patients to seek methamphetamine to feel better. Methamphetamine withdrawal could then lead to further depression and fatigue, and the user might then have sought more methamphetamine to combat those symptoms. Researchers during this period were also learning that long-term, heavy use of methamphetamine was damaging the neuronal brain cells already injured by HIV, leading to cognitive impairments, chronically altered mood states, and persisting psychosis [10].

Although the effects of methamphetamine were being discussed in our clinic's case conferences as if it were a new player on the scene, the drug had been around for a long time. The first known synthesis of methamphetamine from ephedrine was in Japan in 1893, following the formulation of amphetamine in Germany in 1887 [11]. During World War II, branches of the German military used methamphetamine extensively. Eventually physicians in America would recommend amphetamines for weight loss, depression, fatigue, and hyperactive disorders. Cheaper forms of methamphetamine, synthesized in part from 1-phenyl-2-propanone,[20] would become available decades later and called "crank."[21] Production of crank decreased in the 1990s. New methods of synthesis, however, created a more potent drug in larger quantities. This product would be called Ice, Tina, Crystal Meth, or just meth. It could be smoked, slammed,[22] snorted,[23] eaten, or "booty bumped,"[24] and synthesized in garages in small quantities or in remote facilities in larger quantities. Pseudoephedrine, a principal component in the production of meth, was being bought up in increasingly larger quantities from pharmacies [11]. We wondered if the effects we were seeing in the PACE and Stanford Positive Care clinics was limited to our region or if this pattern was nationwide.

Reports from the Arrestee Drug Abuse Monitoring Program showed that three California counties (Sacramento, San Diego, and Santa Clara) consistently ranked among the top five sites nationwide for the percentage of arrestees testing positive for methamphetamine at that time. In 2003, 36.9 % of San Jose adult male arrestees tested positive for methamphetamine at the time of booking [12]. Those male arrestees who admitted to using methamphetamine reported an average of 8.1 days per month of use of the drug [13]. In 2003, amphetamine/methamphetamine accounted for 47 % of adult admission to residential or outpatient treatment facilities in Santa Clara County [12].

---

[20] Also known as P2P and phenylacetone, 1-phenyl-2-propanone is an organic compound with the chemical formula $C_6H_5CH_2CCH_3$.

[21] *Crank* is a term derived from the "crankcase," reportedly where dealers using motorcycles would hide the drug.

[22] *Slammed* refers to intravenous administration.

[23] *Snorted* refers to nasal insufflation.

[24] *Booty bumped* refers to injection into the rectum.

What we were seeing in our clinics reflected the high rate of methamphetamine use in Santa Clara County. New infections could be attributed to meth use, not only in young MSM but also in older men who had practiced safe sex since the beginning of the epidemic and now had been introduced to Tina. For me it was most difficult to see those patients who had survived so much, including discrimination, bullying, rejection, unemployment, and the death of loved ones, now turning to meth. These vulnerable souls were hurting themselves, perhaps recreating familiar situations and feelings.

> "For me it was most difficult to see those patients who had survived so much, including discrimination, bullying, rejection, unemployment, and the death of loved ones, now turning to meth. These vulnerable souls were hurting themselves, perhaps recreating familiar situations and feelings."

Mood disorders were becoming more difficult to treat in those using meth, and some of our patients would ultimately commit suicide. Psychosis resulted, in part, from the surge of dopamine due to the methamphetamine. Antipsychotics were unable to block these dopaminergic tidal waves flooding my patients' synapses. Best practices for treating methamphetamine abuse in the HIV population were still in their infancy. Approaches that held some promise included cognitive behavioral therapy and contingency management.[25] Medications, including some antidepressants and stimulants, were being investigated for their efficacy in reducing the urge to use methamphetamine. We were building a fairly good understanding of methamphetamine, including its effects on dopamine and the nucleus accumbens,[26] and yet we were feeling as vulnerable as our patients. Physicians were demanding evidence-based treatments. We wanted to see our patients thriving. We, however, were seeing our community becoming a public health nightmare.

Joining Forces

"Dr. McGlynn, can you see the patient in Room 1?"

As the only psychiatrist for the PACE and Stanford Positive Care clinics, I was finding work becoming overwhelming, but my passion never wavered. The internists and infectious disease specialists were trained to focus on CD4 counts, HIV viral loads, and the latest antiretroviral medications, so they depended on me to help manage the emotional, behavioral, and cognitive changes they were seeing in their patients. Cases of sexually transmitted diseases and medication nonadherence continued increasing. Physical ailments normally seen in older adults were now affecting younger patients. When the body is in meth-induced sympathetic overdrive, the myocardium can only tolerate so much strain. As a result, ventricular enlargement and heart failure were being seen more and more in meth users of all

---

[25] Contingency management offers reward incentives for negative toxicology screens.

[26] The nucleus accumbens is a region of the basal forebrain involved in pleasure.

ages, leading to permanent disability and loss of a sense of purpose. Chronic dehy-
dration was leading to renal dysfunction and exhaustion. Although science was
conquering HIV, meth was conquering the community. I was feeling completely
impotent. My patients kept coming back to me asking for help, and yet it seemed
that I—we—had nothing to offer.

In 2004 during a staff meeting, I vented my frustration and the need for more
assistance. Our clinics did not have enough money to hire an additional psychiatrist.
My coworkers wanted to help, so we decided to start meeting weekly to discuss
meth and come up with ideas on how to understand the changing community and
what we could do for them. We called ourselves The Crystal Meth Task Force, and the
group included two social workers, a nutritionist, our pharmacist specialist, and me.
After 2 months we were down to four members. The nutritionist dropped out after
another month, stating, "I don't feel like I'm useful here." The remaining social
worker, Niki Stalder-Skarmoutsos, a feisty and energetic young woman, and I
moved forward on our own. I have heard Mozart's String Duo No. 1 for Violin and
Viola in G Major and knew that amazing music could come from just two
instruments. We, however, had no money except for in-kind funding from the PACE
Clinic and realized the only way we were going to make something of our task force
was to get our hands on real money.

Pharmaceutical companies manufacturing antiretroviral medications have made
a concerted effort to help the communities they serve. The first grant we applied for
was from one of the larger companies, and we were awarded $3,000. This seed was
just what we needed to get us motivated to seek out more funding. Santa Clara
County Department of Alcohol and Drug Services (DADS) announced a Request
for Proposals, seeking applications from county-based agencies targeting substance
use in the region. Between the two members of the Crystal Meth Task Force, we
wrote up a thorough proposal.

A crucial element of our application was a solid needs assessment of the county's
LGBT and HIV communities. Unfortunately this was lacking, but we pushed forward without it. We referenced other groups targeting methamphetamine use in San
Francisco, Montana, San Diego, and Los Angeles. At that time, multimedia campaigns were hot, so we decided to use that approach as our platform. We cited the
Montana Meth Project, for example, which had a very moving campaign focusing
on youth at risk. We referenced San Francisco's project targeting the use of meth in
the gay community and their "Dump Tina" campaign. We quoted morbidity and
mortality statistics wherever we could find them. We provided case examples and
how they affected our clinic and community. DADS found it compelling enough to
award us the grant. We now had $225,000 to use over the next 3 years. Our first task
was to build up our group. We reached out to the corrections (Santa Clara County
Main and Elmwood Jails), The Health Trust (community agency including social
workers and nurse case managers working with the HIV population), AIDS Legal
Services, and private HIV providers. We also invited interested consumers. We
understood that the local men's bathhouse was experiencing problems with meth use
in its facility, so we invited its health educator. In the first meeting we filled up the

Table 1.1 Stanford–Santa Clara County Task Force Members

Organization	Number of participants	Credentials (if Applicable)	Interest
Stanford University	5	MD, PsyD candidates	Public health, academic research
Santa Clara Valley Medical Center	3	MD, MSW	Public health
Health Legal Services of Santa Clara County	1–2	JD	Public health, legal services, criminal implications
The Health Trust	5	MSW	Public health, community services
Santa Clara County Public Health Department	2	MPH	Public health, HIV testing
The Watergarden	1	Health Educator	Community impact
Santa Clara County Department of Corrections	1	MD	Criminal implications, public health
Department of Alcohol and Drug Services	3	PhD, MS	Substance abuse services
Community members	15		Public and community health, substance abuse services

room with almost 40 individuals. The meeting was exciting and energized. We had physicians (including one of the internists from the Main Jail), lawyers, social workers, nurses, pharmacists, and community members (Table 1.1). People wanted to be heard. Our initial goals were to create a public awareness campaign for Santa Clara County. We hired a creative consultant and came up with our first logo, which had the theme "Stop, Don't Stop!" capturing the ambivalence of the methamphetamine user. At some point in the midst of presentations, gay pride festivals, and AIDS walks, members voted on a logo and website name change to StopDontStart.org, because our members felt the "don't stop" portion of our first logo sent a mixed message. We created brochures and T-shirts and appeared on local television shows. At the same time, we understood that part of our mission was to educate providers and the community. We developed educational programs and workshops, which we delivered to many organizations, including Planned Parenthood, corrections, public schools, pharmacies, health care agencies, and community centers where those living with HIV gathered. The Santa Clara County Board of Realtors invited us to present at their annual convention, because many landlords were finding their properties being used for the manufacturing of methamphetamine. In order to centralize our programs, we created a website. Two portals were made available, one for providers and the other for community members. The providers' portal offered links and referral information. The consumer/community member portal provided education about methamphetamine and links to find treatment in Santa Clara County.

The newly renamed Stanford–Santa Clara County Methamphetamine Task Force was busy. During our first year of funding, I gave a presentation for a group in San

Bernardino that was also facing huge problems with meth. One of the physician attendees challenged me, saying, "How can you speak here as an expert when you haven't done any meth research yourself?" After my bruises healed, I realized there was a lot of frustration out there and also recognized that we needed to start conducting our own research to understand our particular community. Maggie Chartier, a student in the joint doctoral psychology program between Stanford University School of Medicine and Palo Alto University, had a background in public health and an interest in methamphetamine abuse. She joined our task force and spearheaded a qualitative and quantitative exploration into the community of HIV-positive MSM using methamphetamine. We wanted to understand the motivations for initiation, abstinence, and relapse. We ran focus groups of methamphetamine users and dealers (some participants fulfilled both roles). We began to understand the mindset of our population and were able to share it with others through publications and conference presentations. I was most struck by one of the qualitative findings—that our participants had strong values but that methamphetamine would cause them to compromise those values. I continue to use this theme in therapy with our patients.

Maggie completed her doctoral dissertation based on the research and successfully encouraged other graduate students in the program to continue her work. Our group also explored other factors in methamphetamine abuse, such as the role of hypogonadism.

Having the funding from DADS gave our task force a certain amount of cachet as we applied for other grants, most of which we were successful in obtaining, although none have exceeded $25,000. Nevertheless, we remain grateful for the funding, which allowed us to continue our work. Our latest research was a joint project with the Stanford School of Medicine Division of Infectious Diseases and Geographic Medicine. In this project, we wanted to focus on the acceptability of HIV testing for those at high risk of becoming infected. Most of our previous work focused on the MSM community. In our new endeavor, we wanted to gather data on women and Latino men in San Jose, California. We approached two of the busiest residential treatment facilities in Santa Clara County, Vida Nueva (for Latino men) and Mariposa Lodge (for women), and our project was warmly received. We prepared interactive HIV/Meth educational programs in English and Spanish for the residents. I would present the medical portion, while one of our community members would relate his powerful life story. We conducted pre- and post-testing knowledge assessments that revealed the efficacy of our teaching approach. The findings, however, were sobering. Although the vast majority of the residential clients were being treated for methamphetamine addiction and at high risk for HIV infection, they were not getting tested for the virus. These results has led our task force into new directions, establishing a more solid relationship with the Santa Clara County Department of Public Health, but continuing with our original mission of reducing methamphetamine use and new HIV infections in our region. Sublimation has once again stepped into my life, transforming my feelings of helplessness as a provider to becoming an active community physician.

Outcomes and Effectiveness

Grantors typically, and understandably, request periodic progress reports. Budgets are tedious but those data are tangible and, for the most part, readily available for these reports. Well-defined mission statements, goals, and accomplishments are also easily generated. The task force has received very positive feedback from those who participated in educational programs, focus groups, and community events. But what has been its overall impact? We continue to meet our goals of proposed deliverables. Carefully prepared programs are presented to providers and the community. Our research has been published in peer-reviewed journals and presented at domestic and international conferences. But what about the community impact? The Montana Meth Project (MPP) is the largest task force of its kind and was rated the third most effective philanthropy in Barron's 2010 rankings. Measures of MPP's efficacy, however, have been challenged, although most agree that it has been successful in bringing the dangers of methamphetamine to the consciousness of many regions, both urban and rural. What remains unclear is the public health impact of the MPP's activities. These data represent our challenge as well. There continue to be methamphetamine-related arrests and emergency department presentations in Santa Clara County. Data from 2000 to 2008 present a mixed picture, but methamphetamine continues to dominate substance abuse admissions in Santa Clara County.

The number of new HIV infections has remained constant over the past several years and is largely driven by MSM. A substantial number of newly diagnosed, HIV-positive MSM patients presenting to the PACE Clinic identify sex under the influence of methamphetamine as their main risk factor for acquiring the virus.

Therefore, despite the efforts of the task force, methamphetamine continues to pose a significant public health risk to our community. One cannot help but conclude that the task force's efforts have failed to demonstrate a significant impact on the basis of the numbers presented earlier. Other measures, however, have sustained our energy. Requests for repeat performances and presentations continue to come from schools, community agencies, and clinics locally and from other regions. Based on findings from pre- and post-test evaluations, new medical providers are not receiving sufficient training in medical schools to deal with methamphetamine use disorders. Many are not aware of the connection between methamphetamine and HIV. Community members are coming to our presentations and learning how to understand and find help for friends and family members struggling with methamphetamine addiction. Local high schools have looked to the task force to provide educational programs for youth who may be at risk for using the drug. So although the data indicate an ongoing problem of methamphetamine in the community, those who are on the frontlines as providers and community members continue to view the task force as necessary and relevant. These less tangible data may be what ultimately define our effectiveness, as well as provide the motivation to continue the work that we do.

Conclusion

Transference, a concept notably explored by Sigmund Freud, may be defined as "the redirection of feelings and desires and especially of those unconsciously retained from childhood" [14]. Choosing friends, lovers, and careers may be influenced by positive and negative experiences from childhood, and transference may facilitate this process. As a psychiatrist, I experience very positive feelings when I am sitting with a vulnerable soul who happens to have HIV and feels trapped in the cycle of methamphetamine. All of my patients have HIV and have been hurt in some way at some time; receiving their HIV diagnosis may be just one injury in a long list of others, and they may view the use of meth simply as a way to relieve their pain, even if for a day or two. I want to wrap my arms around these patients and protect them. I want to tell them that they are safe with me and that I will do my best to help them. I want to tell them everything will be okay. Perhaps I am telling myself the same thing as I think about their mortality.

Foucault's writings on leprosy in the Middle Ages could easily apply to HIV/ AIDS in the twentieth and twenty-first centuries. We have seen an illness become known for its medical and cultural implications, while the infected seemingly exist on the fringes of "normal" society. Methamphetamine-use disorders complicate HIV disease and, in the eyes of Foucault, would push its victims even further into the margins of society.

Methamphetamine continues to be produced in large quantities and marketed to the most vulnerable in society, including those with HIV. The Combat Meth Act of 2005, which legislated tougher regulations of products containing ephedrine, pseudoephedrine, and phenylpropanolamine, brought additional awareness about the problem of methamphetamine abuse in the United States. We are reminded that the drug's path of destruction affects us all—from having to produce identification when buying cold products in pharmacies, to seeing our communities experience increasing levels of crime, disease, homelessness, and suffering.

Methamphetamine is a complex medical, public health, and legal challenge that has been present for decades. I believe the role and mission of organizations like the Stanford–Santa Clara County Methamphetamine Task Force will continue to remain relevant in a community affected by methamphetamine and HIV/AIDS. As Foucault reminds us, diseases with medical and cultural implications will leave behind changes that society may not have anticipated. The union of academic and community organizations are essential in the understanding of, and approach to, treating complex diseases. These marriages are especially important when addressing the societal implications, including stigma, behavior, law, and public health. Finally, speaking from my own experience, these organizations provide the means for an individual to transform one's frustration and helplessness into action by mobilizing a group with a shared mission. "Physician, heal thyself."[27]

> "…these organizations provide the means for an individual to transform one's frustration and helplessness into action by mobilizing a group with a shared mission."

---

[27] Luke 4:23.

References

1. Foucault M. Madness and civilization: a history of insanity in the Age of Reason. s.l. New York: Pantheon Books; 1964.
2. Grov C, Golub SA, Parsons JT, Brennan M, Karpiak SE. Loneliness and HIV-related stigma explain depression among older HIV-positive adults. AIDS Care. 2010;22:630–9.
3. Bazell R (Reporter), Brokaw T (Anchor). Early studies on AIDS. *NBC Nightly News,* June 17, 1982. Available at https://archives.nbclearn.com/portal/site/k-12/browse/?cuecard=916. Last accessed 23 Feb 2015.
4. Darnell A, Nance K (Writers), Machine (Performer). There but for the grace of God go I. New York: RCA Victor, 1979.
5. Boynton A. Remembering St. Vincent's. *The New Yorker,* May 17, 2013. Available at http://www.newyorker.com/culture/culture-desk/remembering-st-vincents. Last accessed 23 Feb 2015.
6. France D. Holding AIDS at bay, only to face 'Lazarus Syndrome.' *The New York Times,* October 6, 1998. Available at http://www.nytimes.com/1998/10/06/science/holding-aids-at-bay-only-to-face-lazarus-syndrome.html. Last accessed 23 Feb 2015.
7. O'Brien Q. Methamphetamine use by HIV-positive men. National HIV Prevention Conference. Atlanta: Centers for Disease Control, 2005.
8. Colfax G, Coates TJ, Husnik MJ, Huang Y, Buchbinder S, Koblin B, et al. Longitudinal patterns of methamphetamine, popper (amyl nitrite), and cocaine use and high-risk sexual behavior among a cohort of San Francisco men who have sex with men. J Urban Health. 2005;82: i62–70.
9. Markowitz JC, Kocsis JH, Fishman B, Spielman LA, Jacobsberg LB, Frances AJ. Treatment of depressive symptoms in human immunodeficiency virus-positive patients. Arch Gen Psychiatry. 1998;55:452–7.
10. Chang L, Ernst T, Speck O, Grob CS. Additive effects of HIV and chronic methamphetamine use on brain metabolite abnormalities. Am J Psychiatry. 2005;162:361–9.
11. Yudko E, Murray-Bridges L, Watson-Hauanio S. History of methamphetamine. In: Yudko E, Hall HV, McPherson SB, editors. Methamphetamine use: clinical and forensic aspects. Boca Raton, FL: CRC; 2003. p. 4–10.
12. Department of Alcohol and Drug Services. Treatment admissions and discharges: adult system of care, FY 2003. San Jose, CA: Santa Clara County; 2003.
13. National Institute of Justice. Arrestee Drug Abuse Monitoring Program. Washington DC, National Institute of Justice, 2003.
14. Webster's New Collegiate Dictionary 8th Edition. 1976.

Narrative 2
Building Relationships with At-Risk Populations: A Community Engagement Approach for Longitudinal Research

Helen W. Wilson, Gloria J. Coleman, Brenikki R. Floyd, and Geri R. Donenberg

This is a story of a 15-year community-academic collaboration in Chicago, where work has focused on HIV risk behavior in adolescents. GIRLTALK: We Talk, the latest wave of their study, responds to the disproportionate burdens of violence and sexual health consequences faced by low-income African American girls, with an emphasis on romantic partnerships.

We recently received a call from a participant in our seven-wave longitudinal study. We had not contacted her and were not expecting follow-up at that time. She just called to say hello, to let us know that she had gotten a new job and was doing well. Like many of the young women in our study, finding work was among life's greatest

H.W. Wilson, Ph.D. (✉)
Department of Psychiatry and Behavioral Sciences,
Stanford University School of Medicine, Stanford, CA, USA
e-mail: hwilson3@stanford.edu

G.J. Coleman, B.A., M.S.
Institute of Juvenile Research, Chicago, IL, USA
e-mail: glojc@att.net

B.R. Floyd, Ph.D., M.P.H.
Community Outreach Intervention Projects, School of Public Health,
University of Illinois at Chicago, Chicago, IL, USA
e-mail: brfloyd@uic.edu

G.R. Donenberg, Ph.D.
School of Public Health and College of Medicine,
University of Illinois at Chicago, Chicago, IL, USA
e-mail: gerid@uic.edu

© Springer International Publishing Switzerland 2015
L.W. Roberts et al. (eds.), *Partnerships for Mental Health*,
DOI 10.1007/978-3-319-18884-3_2

challenges. At her last research interview, this young woman had asked if we knew of any job openings. Unfortunately, this is not a service we can provide, but when she did get a job a few months later, she chose to share the good news with us. In moments like this, we realize we have built relationships that impact the lives of these young women in ways that transcend our research protocol. Our participants have come to view the study team as a source of support, and moreover, the success of our longitudinal study is based on these relationships.

This chapter tells a story of how relationships, often immeasurable and unquantifiable, can enhance science in invaluable ways. Our story is not about traditional clinical intervention or community-based participatory research in a strict sense but about how relationships are integral to carrying out successful longitudinal research with hard-to-reach populations. Relationships have allowed us to successfully retain a sample of young women from low-income, underserved communities in Chicago. These women have returned for seven waves of interviews, over more than 10 years, beginning in early adolescence and spanning into emerging adulthood. Over the years, they have been willing to share their stories, revealing sensitive and deeply personal experiences related to sexual behavior and risks, mental health, substance use, trauma, and interpersonal violence.

Introducing the Partners: The Story of Our Collaboration

We begin by describing our relationships and how our collaboration has evolved over the past 15 years (see Fig. 2.1 for a visual chronology). Dr. Wilson's and Dr. Donenberg's partnership began in 1998, when Dr. Wilson began her graduate research at Northwestern University, Feinberg School of Medicine. She was among Dr. Donenberg's first graduate students, and their collaboration has now spanned more than 15 years. Shortly after Dr. Wilson entered the graduate program in clinical psychology, Dr. Donenberg received her first grant for a project examining HIV risk behavior among adolescents in psychiatric treatment, the *Chicago Adolescent Risk and Evaluation Study (CARES)*. Dr. Wilson completed her dissertation work with that project and continued to work with Dr. Donenberg when she moved to the University of Illinois at Chicago (UIC). She took on the role as project director of *CARES*. As a student, Dr. Wilson played a crucial role in writing a new grant to understand mother–daughter relationships and mother–daughter communication in relation to HIV-risk among low-income African American girls, a group we began to recognize as disproportionately burdened by negative health outcomes. This study, later funded by the National Institute of Mental Health, was to become *GIRLTALK*, the focus of this narrative.

Dr. Wilson left Chicago for fellowships on the east coast, where she completed specialized training in child and adolescent trauma and a research fellowship focused on long-term effects of child abuse and neglect. Through this work, she developed an interest in the links between trauma and risk behavior. When Dr. Wilson returned to the Chicago area for her first faculty position, she reconnected

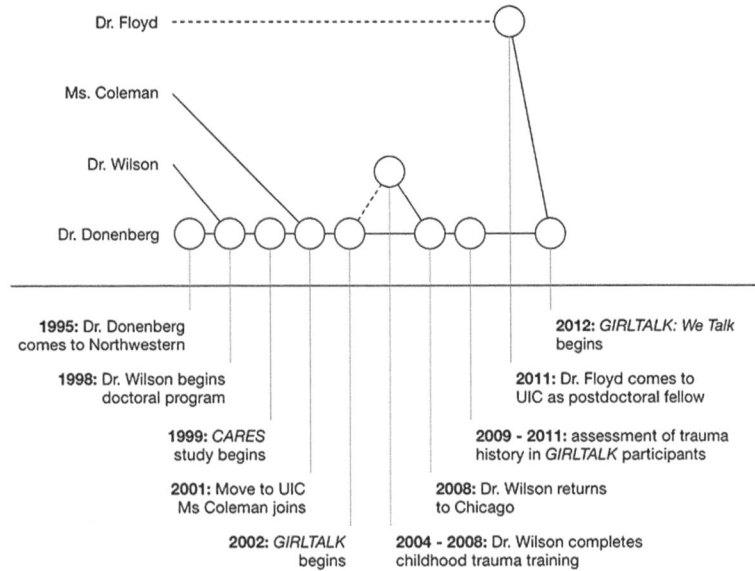

Fig. 2.1 Chronology of the GIRLTALK collaboration

with Dr. Donenberg and the *GIRLTALK* study, and the two renewed their collaboration. Shortly thereafter, Dr. Wilson received her first NIH-funded grant to reinterview the young women from *GIRLTALK* and assess lifetime history of trauma and violence exposure, experiences that had not been adequately explored in the original study. Providers at the original recruitment sites had expressed concerns about high rates of trauma, and Dr. Wilson believed early trauma might play an important role in the development of sexual risk behavior, given that these young women were growing up in neighborhoods with high rates of violence. Over the next few years, the research with *GIRLTALK* shifted to the role of trauma and violence exposure in the development of sexual risk behavior. Dr. Wilson's collaboration with Dr. Donenberg and a research team at UIC including Ms. Coleman and Dr. Floyd allowed her to take a faculty position at Stanford University School of Medicine, from where she continues to lead the *GIRLTALK: We Talk* study.

Ms. Coleman joined the team as the recruitment and tracking coordinator for *CARES* in early 2001, and she brought a wealth of research experience from working with youth and families in the surrounding Chicago areas. She originally came to UIC as a group facilitator and recruiter for a community-based intervention aimed at reducing HIV/AIDS risk in low-income, inner-city African American youth. Shortly after Dr. Donenberg moved to UIC, she met Ms. Coleman and asked her to join our team. She continued to work with us for more than 10 years. Over the course of *GIRLTALK*, Ms. Coleman became a legend with the families; they frequently asked about her at interview appointments and brought her baked goods for the holidays. Dr. Wilson also worked closely with Ms. Coleman on *CARES*, learning much about recruiting and tracking community participants and immediately thought of her as the ideal person to locate and engage the young women in her new study. Because the research team had been out of contact with many of the participants for over 3 years, Ms. Coleman's special touch was crucial for the success of our continued follow-up. Even years after being in contact, she remembered the life stories of many participants and was able to pick up where she left off with them in the new recruitment phase.

After completing her doctoral work at the University of Kentucky, where she was involved with a mass media campaign to encourage adolescents to postpone sexual debut, Dr. Floyd entered a postdoctoral fellowship at UIC with Dr. Donenberg's research team to continue her training with minority populations. Dr. Donenberg introduced her to Dr. Wilson, given their common interests in reducing sexual health risks among adolescent girls. They first worked together in conducting focus groups and interviews in preparation for submitting the revised *GIRLTALK: We Talk* grant proposal. Because of their successful collaboration on this project, Dr. Wilson asked Dr. Floyd to take the role of project director when the grant was funded, and Dr. Floyd has continued to lead data collection for this newest wave of the study.

Defining the Issues

Sexual Risk

Our research focuses on understanding and preventing sexual risk behavior in vulnerable populations. In particular, the *GIRLTALK* study sought to understand the role of mother–daughter relationships and communication in sexual risk taking among African American girls seeking mental health services in low-income Chicago communities. Young African American women are among demographic groups in the United States bearing the highest burden of sexually transmitted infections (STIs), including Human Immunodeficiency Virus (HIV) and Acquired Immune Deficiency Syndrome (AIDS). According to the Centers for Disease Control and Prevention (CDC), HIV/AIDS is the leading cause of death for Black women ages 25–34 years [1], and risk for young Black women is estimated to be 20 times that for young white women [2]. Furthermore, African American women ages 15–24 are the highest risk demographic group for both chlamydia and gonorrhea, according to United States (US) public health department documentation [3]. A nationally representative study with US high school girls reported that 44 % of African American girls, as compared to 20 % of White and Mexican American girls, were infected with an STI [4]. Like other health disparities that affect minority women, disadvantages associated with living in impoverished, underserved communities likely account for disproportionate rates of STIs among young African American women [5]. Furthermore, African American adolescent girls presenting for mental health services represent a particularly vulnerable subgroup in need of effective intervention to reduce risk for STIs. Indeed, youth in psychiatric treatment tend to engage in higher rates of sexual risk behaviors than their peers [6].

Violence Exposure

Violence exposure represents another major public health problem that disproportionately impacts young women growing up in low-income urban neighborhoods [7–11]. Violence exposure is also associated with sexual risk (e.g., [7, 12–16]) and mental health problems [17]. A nationally representative US study found that 60 % of 0 to 17-year-olds experienced physical, sexual, or witnessed violence in the year preceding the study [18]. In another nationally representative study, 48 % of adolescents reported lifetime exposure to violence [19]. Research with youth in Chicago, from similar communities as the *GIRLTALK* women, in the 1990s reported that 26 % of youths aged 7–15 years old had witnessed a shooting, 30 % a stabbing, and 78 % a beating. Half of youth ages 10–19 years old reported physical victimization, and three fourths had witnessed a robbery, stabbing, shooting, or murder. Two thirds of high school students reported being witness to a shooting, nearly one half had witnessed a murder, and over one fourth reported being victims of physical or sexual violence [20, 21]. Given these alarming statistics and links between violence exposure and sexual risk, the newest phase of our work has focused on uncovering pathways from violence exposure to sexual risk in the *GIRLTALK* young women.

Minority Populations: Most Affected, Least Represented

Despite suffering disparate rates of many major health concerns, including violence and sexual risk [5], minority individuals from underserved backgrounds continue to be underrepresented in the published behavioral science literature [22]. In part, this finding relates to the fact that such populations are often hidden, difficult to reach, and distrustful of academic research, making research more costly and challenging to conduct [23]. Yet, research findings with college students or middle-class Caucasians may not generalize to all segments of the population. Moreover, designing effective interventions to reduce health risk requires inclusion of participants from the populations at highest risk. In this narrative, we describe our efforts to maintain a sample of minority women from low-income urban communities.

The Importance and Challenges of Longitudinal Research

Our research uses a longitudinal approach to understand the development of risk behavior and potential risk and protective factors. Most existing research on sexual risk is cross-sectional, correlating reported behavior with reported risk factors, such as early violence exposure. Although cross-sectional studies are cost-effective and play a critical role in the initial stage of establishing a linkage, they represent only a snapshot in development and are unable to capture changes in behavior over time. Examining change over time is particularly important during the dynamic developmental stage of adolescence. Longitudinal data are also critical to understanding phenomena such as sexual behavior, which changes considerably during adolescence and young adulthood. Moreover, longitudinal research allows us to evaluate temporal order of experiences, an essential step in testing causal theories and determining ideal points and targets for intervention.

Despite the benefits of longitudinal research, it comes with a number of challenges [24]. First, this kind of research is undoubtedly an extensive undertaking that requires significant time and resources. Second, individuals who participate in longitudinal research may be unique from their peers, given the commitment required over multiple years and assessments. Third, it is possible that variables most relevant for the individuals in a longitudinal study are no longer the most significant for later generations, making results obscure by the time findings are published. Fourth, the most significant challenge of longitudinal research is perhaps attrition, which is the primary focus of this narrative.

Over the waves of a longitudinal study, participants are inevitably lost, and if attrition is high or selects for important characteristics (e.g., the highest risk or lowest risk individuals drop out at higher rates than others), findings can be biased in important ways. Thus, two of the most challenging and critical aspects of longitudinal research are reducing attrition and, when there is attrition, reducing systematic loss of participants with particular characteristics. In research with low-income, urban minority populations, these issues can be particularly challenging due to high mobility [25, 26]. The hardest-to-reach participants may be those with the most chaotic and difficult life circumstances, such as homelessness, and it is crucial that such individuals continue to be represented. This narrative describes how our relationships with the study participants have played an integral role in maintaining the sample and enhancing the success of the project.

The *GIRLTALK* Study

GIRLTALK is a longitudinal study that originally focused on mother–daughter relationships, mother–daughter communication, and peer and partner relationships as predictors of HIV-risk behavior among African American girls recruited from mental health agencies serving low-income communities in Chicago. The girls entered the study at ages 12–16 (average age 14). They were followed for 2 years and completed five interviews until they were ages 14–18 (average age 16). Recognizing the high rates of violence in the communities where the girls resided and the potential role of violence in risk behavior, a sixth interview at average age 17 focused on a comprehensive assessment of trauma and violence exposure, including physical, sexual, and witnessed violence. It became clear from the interviews that many girls had experienced violence in their romantic relationships, and violence involving dating partners was strongly associated with sexual risk. These findings led to the current wave of data collection addressing romantic partnerships, including partner violence, as women are entering adulthood (ages 18–25). We call this newest wave *GIRLTALK: We Talk* to highlight the focus on couples and dyadic relationships. Thus, relationships, first with mothers and now with partners, are central to the design of the study itself.

Embarking on this research initially involved forming relationships with community agencies and stakeholders at the mental health agencies where we identified and recruited adolescent girls and their mothers. Early in the process, we elicited input from community members to refine our questions, measures, and procedures, through focus groups, community advisory board meetings, and pilot testing. Our advisory board met annually and was integral to understanding some of the emerging trends and findings. But this story focuses primarily on the relationships we have developed with the participants themselves.

> *"… relationships, first with mothers and now with partners, are central to the design of the study itself."*

Over the first five waves of the study, we successfully retained 76–81 % of the baseline sample of 266 mother–daughter dyads. At the sixth wave, we only invited girls who participated in at least one of the five follow-up interviews. We enrolled 74 % of those who were eligible (177 out of 239), although more than a year had passed on average since the last contact, and several years had passed for many participants. Of the 177 girls who participated in Wave 6, we have so far interviewed 123 women in *GIRLTALK: We Talk*, and recruitment efforts are still underway with plans to enroll 130–150. We are also recruiting the young women's romantic or sexual partners to participate. Although attrition is a risk and limitation of longitudinal research, we see our ability to remain in contact with these women as a success story. Nonetheless, we have lost a proportion of the women at each follow-up and are now facing the challenge of recruiting the most hard-to-reach participants in the sample. Predictably, over the past 10 years, the *GIRLTALK* women have regularly moved and changed their phone numbers, and we have had to rely on multiple contacts and chains of contact with collateral friends, family members, and community members such as pastors. In many cases, we have reached what may be dead-ends with letters returned and all available phone numbers disconnected. Next steps include going into the field and knocking on doors at the last-known residences and using online people searches. Despite these challenges, we believe our efforts to follow the women from early adolescence to emerging adulthood are worth the ability to capture developmental changes in a way that is lost in studies relying on cross-sectional designs.

The Role of Relationships in Retaining Participants

In preparing for *GIRLTALK: We Talk*, we mailed letters to all of the young women who participated in the sixth wave of data collection to notify them that a new study would be launching for which they may be eligible. A few months later, we received a message from a staff member in the UIC department where the original waves of the study took place (the project had moved to a new department in a new building). A woman had come to the university looking for the *GIRLTALK* study. It turned out that she was the mother of a participant who had received our letter, but before she could contact us or pass the information on to her daughter, the letter was lost in a house fire. And yet she recalled the letter and wanted to make sure that her daughter could participate again.

How is it that we have been able to retain this sample, with the dedication of participants exhibited by the story above? In short, trust, genuine concern, and consistent respect for each individual family's life story. Scientifically, we have employed a number of incentives and tracking procedures found to be successful in longitudinal research [27, 28]. We provide gifts after each interview, such as T-shirts, key chains, and water bottles with the study logo. During the initial five waves, we called families monthly to update their locator information, and we began contacting families several months before the newest wave of funding came through, in anticipation of the project. We sent birthday cards with movie passes, holiday cards, and postcards with return addresses so that families could update us if they moved. We continue to send newsletters summarizing findings from *GIRLTALK* and related information and resources. Although these strategies undoubtedly help, we believe it is something more, something less tangible that has motivated these women to keep returning.

Relationships in the Context of Recruitment and Tracking

Including Community Members on the Recruitment Team

One critical way that we have maintained relationships with the women is in the context of recruitment and tracking. Our recruitment team includes individuals from the same or similar communities where the young women live. At times, recruiters may even encounter participants in the community. This situation can of course raise challenges. We learned that one of our recruiters, approximately the same age as the women at the current wave, went to the same high school as some of our participants. Although the situation was helpful in the recruiter being able to relate to the participants, we have had to take extra precautions regarding confidentiality. The recruiter was advised to be conscious of the similarities she has with the participants and their curiosity about her position on the research team because participants have sometimes asked her about finding similar work. We asked her to limit conversation around her personal and educational background and to redirect questions about her age, full name, or where she grew up and went to school.

Mindful of issues such as confidentially, coercion, or dual relationships, we have used community connections to build relationships. Once, at a dinner at her church, someone at the table recognized Ms. Coleman's voice. It turned out she was a participant whom Ms. Coleman had tried to contact several times. The participant had lost our number, and we had not reached her. After this encounter, Ms. Coleman was able to schedule her assessment, and she completed the study. When recruiters go into the field to knock on doors, most people cautiously crack the door, seeming understandably wary at first. But when the recruiters mention *GIRLTALK*, they are usually greeted warmly invited to come inside.

An Approach that Blends Warmth and Persistence

Our recruitment approach blends warmth with persistence and recognizes that participants face numerous stressors that often take priority over participating in research. Many of the young women enrolled in our studies are in school, working, and/or raising children. Unemployment is often a serious concern that makes basic survival paramount. So when attempting to recruit these women, we are not thwarted by hang-ups, an impolite response from an individual answering the phone, or a no-show to a scheduled interview. We assume these events are not personal but, rather, that the individual is focused on other important matters that take precedence. Often, they are simply unable to think about the study at that moment. We sometimes reach a family member who does not know about the study or reacts negatively. We have found it important not to let such interactions negatively affect us. We just call back later, until we get someone else on the phone or reach the participant at a better time. While persistent, we are always friendly and, without pushing, might say something like, "I'm not trying to bug you, and if you've got other things to do it's fine, just let me know a good time to call you back." We respond to hang-ups by calling back and politely saying something like, "I believe we got disconnected" or "I'm sorry. I think I hung up on you."

We have also learned to be flexible by calling participants at various times of day, including evenings and weekends, and asking what times are best to reach them. We make every effort to call at times convenient to the participant, which could be 10:00 at night or on a Sunday afternoon. We recognize that our participants are individuals with many other priorities, and we convey that we value their time. To enhance our recruitment efforts, we have incorporated various modes of communication, such as text messages and voice calls, and ask participants the best means to reach them. We have found that many participants avoid answering an unrecognized number and respond more quickly to a text message than a voicemail. Of course, we are respectful if a participant indicates that she no longer wants contact from us, although we have rarely had this response.

At times life will get in the way of participation, but young women who have benefited from our previous research typically find ways around life's challenges to continue their involvement. Participants sometimes express interest in participating but ask to be contacted at a later time. For example, one young woman scheduled for a *GIRLTALK: We Talk* interview did not attend her scheduled appointment. After multiple attempts to contact her to reschedule, she eventually explained that she was dealing with some personal issues and asked if we would call her in a couple of months to schedule another interview. In some cases, we have scheduled recruitment calls to take place during specific times of the year due to a participant's request. For instance, another young woman was in the process of planning her summer wedding and asked us to call her back at the beginning of the fall. She wanted to participate but could not make time for the study at the time we called due to this important life event.

A number of our participants are away at school or have relocated out of Chicago, sometimes out of the state. Some of these out-of-town participants schedule interviews when they return to Chicago, even if it means giving up time with friends and family. Others do not plan to visit Chicago, and we travel to their location to interview them. Participants who are initially hesitant to participate have brightened in tone and eagerly accepted when we offered to travel to them. One recent out-of-town participant expressed, "This study must be really important if you're willing to come all the way to me," and others have made similar statements.

Treating Participants as Humans, Rather Than Numbers

Our recruitment team takes genuine interest in the lives and experiences of our participants and treats them as people rather than merely research subjects we are trying to recruit. We have found that conveying interest in and showing care for what is going on in their lives goes a long way. Similarly, we find that people tend to warm up when they realize we have their interests at heart. Thus, recruiters pay attention to important events, such as birthdays, surgeries, weddings, childbirths, and family illnesses and deaths. We listen to the young women when they want to talk about their wedding plans or job searches. We are mindful of life events when we contact participants and make sure to ask about them when we do make contact. These personal touches make a difference. When participants arrive for their interviews, they usually ask to see "Miss Gloria" or other individuals who have been involved in recruitment. At the end of an interview, we often spend additional time talking with the women. Many ask about future opportunities to participate in our research studies or inquire of ways their friends or family members could get involved. We believe the young women and their mothers have learned that we genuinely care about them, and some families have said they would participate even if we offered no compensation.

Relationships Through Giving Something Back

Maximizing Benefits

Another critical aspect of our relationships with the participants involves giving back to the community, or at least to the young women participating in our study. *GIRLTALK* mothers often told us that they continued to participate because they felt the study benefitted their daughters, themselves, and their relationship. They particularly enjoyed a part of the study that involved mothers and daughters discussing a conflict in their relationship and trying to resolve the problem. The families appreciated the attention they received from the project staff. Although there was no active intervention, the mothers frequently shared that they felt "better" and that their daughters were "better" because they participated in *GIRLTALK*. This experience was shared by a participant in *GIRLTALK: We Talk* who expressed how much she and her mother benefited from being in the previous *GIRLTALK* study. She told us that before *GIRLTALK* she did not have a relationship with her mother, but after participating in the study, their relationship improved greatly—so much so that she relocated to be closer to her mother, and their communication remains positive today.

Similarly, the young women in *GIRLTALK: We Talk* tell us they have gained from thinking about their romantic relationships and participating with their partners. Many of the women have said it was helpful to participate in a videotaped interaction during which they discuss actual relationship conflicts with a romantic partner. Some participants have shared how helpful it was to talk with their partners about real relationship issues because they rarely have the opportunity to talk about these kinds of concerns. For some couples, this may be an opportunity to face topics they are avoiding. During a follow-up call, one couple told us that they decided to break up after airing conflicts during the videotaped interaction but were able to work things out and later got back together. As with the mothers and daughters, couples appear to benefit from discussing these issues in a safe, structured setting. A number of the young women and their partners have also said they enjoyed this activity as a way to help other women and couples. At the end of the partner interview, several couples have described plans to use their study compensation for a date night, and we have noticed numerous couples leave the study holding hands.

Providing Support and Referrals

Another way in which the project gives back is through careful attention to women's safety and security. At the end of each interview, we provide referrals for mental health services and other resources if concerns such as suicidal ideation, intimate partner violence, or abuse arise, or if requested by participants. When women report relationship violence or suicidal ideation during the interview, we assess their risk

of harm and help them develop safety plans. As a standard, we give everyone information about healthy relationships, recognizing when relationships are abusive, and
referrals for domestic violence services including shelters, legal advocacy, and
obtaining protective orders. We also offer to help link them with a service if desired.
When a participant came to her *GIRLTALK: We Talk* appointment with a fresh black
eye and limping, we were immediately concerned. During the interview, she
revealed that she had been assaulted a few days earlier by members of her ex-
boyfriend's gang. We were able to provide her with a confidential hotline number
through the Chicago Police Department for reporting gang-related incidents. In
addition, she had not sought medical attention and accepted with appreciation our
offer to walk her to the university medical center emergency department.

   Although our study is not an intervention, we believe that many young women
return because they feel connected to our staff, value the relationships that we continue to nurture, and have gained something meaningful from being a part of the
study. This kind of relationship can also bring about challenges when participants
need services we cannot provide but see our site as a safe, trusted place. When we
contacted one participant to schedule her appointment with her romantic partner,
she disclosed that she was experiencing abuse from her live-in boyfriend and needed
help. She did not want us to call the police out of fear of negative consequences
from her landlord. Instead, the young woman asked to come to our lab at UIC, over
an hour away from where she lived. While respecting the participant's wish not to
involve the police, we assessed her immediate safety over the phone and kept her on
the line while identifying and contacting domestic violence shelters in her community. Although we could not provide these services directly, we were able to convince her to meet with a local domestic violence advocate who would be in a better
position to help her.

   From a purely scientific perspective, one could argue that this kind of relationship changes the participants' experience and access to services, and therefore
threatens the validity of our findings. In clinical research, there are always important
tradeoffs and balances to weigh. In this case, we strongly believe that in recruiting
vulnerable, underserved populations such as these young women, the scientific
costs are worth it. As they are willing to share deeply personal information, revealing experiences such as abuse and intimate partner violence, for the sake of our
scientific endeavor, it is our ethical and moral obligation to provide something in
return. And as this chapter emphasizes, these efforts to support and maintain positive relationships with the sample have enhanced the science in numerous ways.

Integrating a Service

In *GIRLTALK: We Talk*, we are able to offer an even more direct and tangible benefit
to participants through tests and treatment for STIs. Scientifically, we are interested
in conducting biological tests for STIs as an objective indicator of sexual risk. This
choice also brings up an ethical obligation, however. Because most STIs are non-
symptomatic, it is common for individuals to be unaware that they are infected.

Moreover, many of the women in our study lack consistent health care. Untreated STIs can lead to negative health outcomes for individuals and have serious implications for public health. Thus, in designing this wave of the study we felt ethically obligated to provide treatment for participants who tested positive. To do this, we looked to intervention studies being conducted by Dr. Donenberg's lab that provided testing and treatment for STIs. We decided to use the same procedures, even though our study is not intended to be an intervention.

We test each woman and her partner for three STIs—chlamydia, gonorrhea, and trichomoniasis—that can be tested relatively non-invasively with urine samples. We notify all participants of their results, whether positive or negative. For those who test positive, we offer no-cost treatment and counseling from a physician who is part of the study team. We coordinate these appointments and escort participants to the doctor's office. We also offer transportation to the appointment. Thus far, 30 % of the women and 11 % of their partners have tested positive for at least one STI. Over half (54 %) have chosen to see our doctor, and an additional 33 % told us they received appropriate treatment from their personal doctor. A particularly meaningful experience occurred when both members of a couple tested positive and chose to schedule their treatment and counseling together. We were able to transport the couple to an appointment with the study doctor. While biological tests for STIs meet a scientific aim of the study in providing objective data demonstrating risk, these procedures also allow us to offer participants a valuable intervention and service.

As well as enhancing relationships with the participants and fulfilling what we believe is our ethical obligation, this kind of intervention offers a different approach than much traditional research. Over the history of clinical research, underserved populations have often been exploited—horrific examples such as the Tuskegee Syphilis experiment come to mind. We tend to think of these kinds of transgressions as artifacts of the past, but HIV/AIDS research as recently as the 2000s has been plagued with controversies around withholding of treatment [29]. Although we are not engaged in community participatory research to develop an intervention per se, we provide support and assistance in getting treatment for those who reveal clinical concerns. Thus, in addition to benefitting individual participants, these actions may help to foster greater trust in research institutions [30]. Our work is associated with the *Community Outreach Intervention Projects* (COIP), a public health program within the UIC School of Public Health that has been involved with the community for over 25 years, providing much needed medical care and other services to individuals from low-income communities of Chicago and integrating research and interventions to reduce HIV/AIDS.

What Have We Learned?

The ultimate goal of our research is to inform the design of intervention and prevention efforts to reduce risk for problems such as STIs and intimate partner violence among women who are disproportionately affected by these problems. With longitudinal data, we are able to identify risk markers, protective factors, and health outcomes across different stages of development. For example, we have found that in early adolescence, girls' sexual experience was associated with externalizing problems (e.g., aggression, delinquency), more permissive parenting, less open mother–daughter sexual communication, and more frequent mother–daughter communication [31]. Among sexually active girls, mother–daughter attachment was associated with more consistent condom use [31]. Other findings suggest that family and peer relationships work together to influence sexual risk. Stronger mother–daughter attachment was associated with having less risky peers, which was in turn linked to less sexual risk behavior self-reported by the girls [32]. Results from the original *GIRLTALK* waves formed the basis for a mother–daughter intervention to reduce HIV risk, which is currently being evaluated in a randomized clinical trial with girls from the same low-income communities in Chicago.

Incorporating Wave 6 data, we are now examining the role of violence exposure in the development of sexual risk behavior. So far, we have found that violence exposure during childhood was associated with increased likelihood of sexual activity in early adolescence, but only risk behaviors (e.g., inconsistent condom use and multiple partners) during late adolescence when sexual activity is normative [33]. We have also found that violence in the context of romantic relationships, as compared to relationships with family members, peers, or other community members, is most strongly associated with sexual risk in our sample [7]. These findings led to the development of the *GIRLTALK: We Talk* study focused on romantic relationships. Dr. Wilson is now designing an intervention that combines elements of empirically supported interventions for trauma, HIV risk, and dating violence to promote healthy romantic relationships in girls with histories of violence exposure.

Recommendations for Building Relationships in Longitudinal Research

Our experience with this longitudinal study with young women in Chicago has provided us with a unique perspective, which we hope will be helpful for other researchers. We have learned a number of lessons that may be useful for research teams who wish to conduct similar research that involves following hard-to-reach populations over time. First, it is essential to develop strong relationships with community stakeholders and representatives during the initial stages of the research design and plans. Second, we have found it to be extremely beneficial to select recruiters and assemble recruitment teams who have backgrounds and experiences that reflect those of the participant population. Third, a recruitment approach blending warmth and persistence is most effective. It is helpful for recruiters to maintain a "thick skin" so that they remain positive, friendly, and persistent despite inevitable rejection and difficulty finding participants. It is equally important that the recruiter treats each participant as a unique individual and takes interest in participants' lives, noting the best times to reach them and remembering important life events. Fourth, we suggest that finding ways to directly benefit participants in longitudinal research is not only an ethical obligation but also enhances relationships and retention. Beyond enhancing science and fulfilling our ethical obligations, we have found that this approach and the relationships built make the work particularly meaningful for our research team.

Adequate representation of ethnic and racial minorities in research is essential for reducing health disparities in the USA, and effective recruitment and retention is necessary for adequate representation. Other researchers have found that strategies incorporating community involvement, in person contact, telephone follow-up, and timely incentives are likely to be most effective in recruiting and retaining minority participants [34]. Although it takes considerable effort, time, and resources, the cultivation of these approaches has proven effective in building trust and rapport with a sample of low-income African American young women, thereby allowing us to follow them from adolescence into young adulthood and now helping us to recruit their romantic partners. In order to carry out this work, we have relied on strong collaborative relationships within our research team that have evolved over more than a decade. Our partnership continues to build on past successes and the unique experiences and strengths of each team member.

Conclusion

Building relationships with our participants has been central to the success of our research following a longitudinal sample of young African American women from low-income communities in Chicago. Through their continued participation, we are gaining valuable knowledge for designing effective interventions to reduce significant public health problems, such as STIs and intimate partner violence, which disproportionately affect low-income minority women. The young women of the *GIRLTALK* study have gifted us with their time, dedication, and life stories. Although we have only looked into a small window of their lives, the stories they have been willing to share mean much more than a data point.

References

1. Centers for Disease Control and Prevention. HIV/AIDS among women. CDC HIV/AIDS Fact Sheet 2008.
2. Centers for Disease Control and Prevention. CDC Fact Sheet: HIV among African American youth. 2014.
3. Centers for Disease Control and Prevention. Sexually transmitted disease surveillance 2011. Atlanta, GA: U.S. Department of Health and Human Services; 2012.
4. Forhan SE, Gottlieb SL, Sternberg MR, Xu F, Datta SD, McQuillan GM, et al. Prevalence of sexually transmitted infections among female adolescents aged 14 to 19 in the United States. Pediatrics. 2009;124:1505–12.

5. Pearlin L, Schieman S, Fazio EM, Meersman SC. Stress, health, and the life course: some conceptual perspectives. J Health Soc Behav. 2005;46:205–19.
6. Donenberg GR, Pao M. HIV/AIDS prevention and intervention: youths and psychiatric illness. Contemp Psychiatry. 2004;2:1–8.
7. Wilson HW, Woods BA, Emerson E, Donenberg GR. Patterns of violence exposure and sexual risk in low-income, urban African American girls. Psychol Violence. 2012;2:194–207.
8. Foster H, Brooks-Gunn J, Martin A, Flannery DJ, Vazsonyi AT, Waldman ID. Poverty/socioeconomic status and exposure to violence in the lives of children and adolescents. The Cambridge handbook of violent behavior and aggression. New York, NY: Cambridge University Press; 2007. p. 664–87.
9. Voisin DR. The effects of family and community violence exposure among youth: recommendations for practice and policy. J Soc Work Educ. 2007;43:51–66.
10. Berman SL, Silverman WK, Kurtines WM. The effects of community violence on children and adolescents: intervention and social policy. In: Bottoms BL, Kovera MB, McAuliff BD, editors. Children, social science, and the law. Cambridge, UK: Cambridge University Press; 2002. p. 301–21.
11. Osofsky JD. The impact of violence on children. Domest Violence Child. 1999;9(3):33–49.
12. Voisin DR, Neilands TB. Community violence and health risk factors among adolescents among adolescents on Chicago's Southside: does gender matter? J Adolesc Health. 2010;46:600–2.
13. Brady SS, Donenberg GR. Mechanisms linking violence exposure to health risk behavior in adolescence: motivation to cope and sensation seeking. J Am Acad Child Adolesc Psychiatry. 2006;45:673–80.
14. Wyatt GE, Myers HF, Williams JK, Kitchen CR, Loeb T, Carmona JV, et al. Does a history of trauma contribute to HIV risk for women of color? Implications for prevention and policy. Am J Public Health. 2002;92:660–5.
15. Wilson HW, Widom CS. An examination of risky sexual behavior and HIV among victims of child abuse and neglect: a thirty-year follow-up. Health Psychol. 2008;27:49–158.
16. Senn TE, Carey MP, Vanable PA. Childhood and adolescent sexual abuse and subsequent sexual risk behavior: evidence from controlled studies, methodological critique, and suggestions for research. Clin Psychol Rev. 2008;28:711–35.
17. McDonald CC, Richmond TR. The relationship between community violence exposure and mental health symptoms in urban adolescents. J Psychiatr Ment Health Nurs. 2008;15: 833–49.
18. Finkelhor D, Turner HA, Ormrod RK, Hamby SL. Violence, abuse, and crime exposure in a national sample of children and youth. Pediatrics. 2009;124:1411–23.
19. Hanson RF, Borntrager C, Self-Brown S, Kilpatrick DG, Saunders BE, Resnick HS, et al. Relations among gender, violence exposure, and mental health: The National Survey of Adolescents. Am J Orthopsychiatry. 2008;78:313–21.
20. Jenkins EJ, Bell CC. Violence among inner city high school students and post-traumatic stress disorder. In: Friedman S, editor. Anxiety disorders in African Americans. New York: Springer; 1994. p. 76–88.
21. Bell CC, Jenkins EJ. Community violence and children on Chicago's Southside. Psychiatry. 1993;56(1):46–54.
22. Arnett JJ. The neglected 95%: why American psychology needs to become less American. Am Psychol. 2008;63(7):602–14.
23. Sue S. Science, ethnicity, and bias: where have we gone wrong? Am Psychol. 1999;54(12): 1070–7.
24. Lerner RM. Methodological issues in the study of human development concepts and theories of human development. Lawrence Erlbaum Associates, Inc.; 2002. p. 480–517.
25. Lewis DA, Sinha V. Moving up and moving out? Economic and residential mobility of low-income Chicago families. Urban Aff Rev. 2007;43.
26. Jelleyman T, Spencer N. Residential mobility in childhood and health outcomes: a systematic review. J Epidemiol Community Health. 2008;62:584–92.

27. Blachman DR, Esposito L. Getting started: answering your frequently asked questions about applied research on child and adolescent development. In: Maholmes V, Lomonaco CG, editors. Applied research in child and adolescent development: a practical guide. New York, NY: Psychology Press; 2010. p. 7–37.
28. Kapungu CT, Nappi CM, Thakral C, Miller SA, Devlin C, McBride C, et al. Recruiting and retaining high-risk HIV adolescents into family-based HIV prevention intervention research. J Child Fam Stud. 2012;21(4):578–88.
29. Kazdin AE. Ethical issues and guidelines for research. Research design in clinical psychology. Boston: Allyn and Bacon; 2003.
30. Smith MB. Moral foundations in research with human participants. In: Sales BD, Folkman S, editors. Ethics in research with human participants. Washington, DC: American Psychological Association; 2000.
31. Donenberg GR, Emerson E, Mackesy-Amiti ME. Sexual risk among African American girls: psychopathology and mother–daughter relationships. J Consult Clin Psychol. 2011;79(2): 153–8.
32. Emerson E, Donenberg GR, Wilson HW. Health-protective effects of attachment among African American girls in psychiatric care. J Fam Psychol. 2012;26(1):124–32.
33. Wilson HW, Donenberg GR, Emerson E. Childhood violence exposure and the development of sexual risk in low-income African American girls. J Behav Med. 2014;37:1091–101.
34. Yancey AK, Ortega AN, Kumanyika SK. Effective recruitment and retention of minority research participants. Annu Rev Public Health. 2006;27(1):1–28.

Narrative 3
The Center for Youth Wellness: A Community-Based Approach to Holistic Health Care in San Francisco

Suzanne E. Walker and Victor G. Carrion

This is a story that chronicles the convening of multiple academic and community stakeholders in San Francisco to create a trauma-informed system of care by collocating three organizations to address the adversity that children and youth living in poverty face daily.

Central Moment

Beginning in 2007, practitioners from around the Bay Area of California came together to have informal conversations about how to address the ongoing issue of toxic stress and trauma that children and youth in San Francisco face on a daily basis. We define toxic stress here as resulting from "strong, frequent, or prolonged activation of the body's stress response systems," impacting the brain and other physiological responses to stress [1]. Knowing that exposure to this type of stress—stemming from abuse, neglect, witnessing community or interpersonal violence, and the challenges of growing up in poverty—had deleterious effects on individuals' health and well-being, we formed a multidisciplinary group determined to create a coordinated approach to the issue. Our partnership was made up of an unlikely

S.E. Walker, M.A. (✉)
San Francisco State University, San Francisco, CA, USA
e-mail: swalker@mail.sfsu.edu

V.G. Carrion, M.D.
Department of Psychiatry and Behavioral Sciences, Stanford University School of Medicine and Lucile Packard Children's Hospital, Stanford, CA, USA
e-mail: vcarrion@stanford.edu

© Springer International Publishing Switzerland 2015
L.W. Roberts et al. (eds.), *Partnerships for Mental Health*,
DOI 10.1007/978-3-319-18884-3_3

group of researchers, health practitioners, child abuse prevention specialists, and other service providers whose work focused on alleviating poverty or improving juvenile justice systems. In traditional health care models, these various practitioners and advocates work separately, often focused on similar, overlapping systemic problems. We wanted to bring together voices across disciplinary lines to address this complex reality.

After narrowing in on the problem of early childhood stress and its associated conditions, the central question in our group became whether to (1) integrate services under one organization, (2) refer patients across various coordinated providers, or (3) collocate separate partners under one roof. We knew that such a complex issue needed a variety of coordinated services, innovative care, and sustainability. Originally we conceived of the Center for Youth Wellness as a single entity, with three main partner organizations sharing the Center for Youth Wellness identity. This arrangement, however, proved to work against the aim of the model—to provide trauma-informed, holistic, and innovative care to patients and families experiencing chronic stress and trauma. Given the intricacies and power of each suborganization's work, an urgent timeline to get services to families, and the need for enough funding for essential programs in a competitive environment, the arrangement of a fully integrated, one-organization model threatened the possibility of no Center for Youth Wellness at all.

Ultimately, we decided upon a collocated approach, which has allowed the partner organizations to maximize their areas of expertise while coordinating care in one accessible location for families. They are able to independently and fully implement programs that serve their respective missions while retaining the opportunity to work collaboratively with one another in service of the community. Now, three organizations are collocated in the Center for Youth Wellness building, offering pediatric, mental health, child abuse prevention, and wellness programming for children and families in the Bayview Hunters Point neighborhood of San Francisco.

Defining the Issue

Chronic stress and trauma affect an extensive number of people across the country. Whether due to interpersonal, community, or institutional violence, the heightened strain that comes with living in poverty, such as the insecurity of one's ability to put food on the table or find safe housing, or experiencing daily microaggressions and decreased opportunity as a person of color in an institutionally racist society, we knew that ongoing stress negatively impacts mental and physiological health. Particularly for children and youth, the results of enduring such chronic adversity may follow them throughout their lives in the form of academic challenges, long-term health conditions such as asthma or diabetes, or anxiety and depression.

In the United States, for example, children and youth are exposed to extraordinary rates of violence. In 2010, among youth aged 15–24 years old, homicide was the second highest cause of death generally and, in particular, the number one reason for death for African Americans, second for Latinos, and third for American Indians and Alaska Natives aged 10–24 years old [2].

Traditional responses to such widespread conditions have their own set of challenges and limitations, among which include lack of financial opportunities. For example, funding for community health centers has continuously declined for over the past 4 or more years [3]. Additionally, researchers have identified a lack of evidence-based interventions in approaches for early childhood interventions and youth psychology [4, 5].

Among resource-scarce communities in urban areas there is a great need for accessible, community-based, and coordinated care to support children and their families. Research has shown a strong connection between urban planning and public health disparities, citing segregation and other social or physical environment factors in urban areas leading to health inequalities, such as housing, mobility, and other factors traditionally placed solely in the social domain [5, 6]. An example of such a community, Bayview Hunters Point was our center site to develop and implement a trauma-informed, one-stop, integrative model working to address not only individual but also family, community, and social needs.

Bayview Hunters Point is a long-standing residential neighborhood of San Francisco that has experienced high rates of poverty, community violence, and toxic environmental exposure. Historically an African American neighborhood, Bayview has experienced a significant amount of adversity from economic challenges, lack of quality housing and healthy food options, institutionalized racism and isolation from the remainder of San Francisco, and exposure to environmental toxins left behind when the Hunters Point Shipyard and power plant closed [7]. As a result, Bayview residents experience much higher rates of chronic illnesses like diabetes, asthma hospitalization rates [7], ischemic heart disease, cancer, and other cardiovascular illnesses. Violence, however, is the number one cause of lives lost in Bayview Hunters Point [8]. Given these factors, we saw a need for a holistic approach to health care in the neighborhood, one that addressed health outcomes stemming from seemingly nonmedical factors.

Researchers have been calling for the expansion of clinical medicine into the social space for some time. An example of this is the difference between a "medical home" and "health neighborhood" [9]. By creating health neighborhoods, which utilize "community-based, nonmedical services that promote the health of patients and families" and incorporate the "identification of basic needs and facilitation of referrals, care coordination, co-location, and centralization of services" [9], health care providers support the whole person, the whole family, and the whole community. Doing so, however, requires multiple stakeholders offering different services to partner in order to support individuals, families, and entire communities.

Specifically, federally qualified health centers act as a "safety net provider" [10] in underresourced communities and offer primary care, housing, or other services. Often known as community health centers, they must fit the following requirements to be federally qualified: (1) retain private nonprofit or public organization status; (2) offer extensive primary care services; (3) offer services to low-income communities with limited access to resources; (4) provide sliding fee scale to uninsured patients; and (5) obtain an independent and community-based board of directors [11].

Reflecting national approaches, health services in San Francisco and the greater Bay Area have traditionally focused on clinical disease only [12], not the issues that were deemed social problems, such as exposure to violence or scarce housing, leading to a lack of resources in the clinical space devoted to addressing social inequities. Because these challenges exist in both the traditional health care and other social settings, such as schools, there is a need to combine these sectors to effectively target the problem [12]. In developing the Center in Bayview Hunters Point, it became critical to work with stakeholders around the community, such as juvenile justice and other community-based public service providers, in order to scale interventions from individuals and families to the community systems level.

The Center for Youth Wellness is a collocated pediatric and mental health care model in Bayview Hunters Point. Made up of a number of partners from different spheres of the nonprofit and public sectors, the Center for Youth Wellness is an approach to address the high prevalence of adversity that children and youth, especially those living in poverty, face in the southeast sector of San Francisco. Low-income families and communities of color in the city experience ongoing toxic stress and trauma due to a multitude of external stressors. Specifically, the Center for Youth Wellness utilizes the Adverse Childhood Experiences (ACEs) diagnostic tool, derived from the renowned Kaiser ACEs study [13], to understand how patients experience toxic stress.

For some background context, the Kaiser ACEs study showed a dose–response relationship between exposure to ACEs and adult risk of chronic disease [13]. The ACEs categories include (1) physical abuse; (2) emotional abuse; (3) contact sexual abuse; (4) physical neglect; (5) emotional neglect; (6) someone chronically depressed, mentally ill, institutionalized, or suicidal; (7) mother treated violently; (8) one or no parents, parental separation, or divorce; and (9) substance abuse in the household [14]. One of the central findings of the ACEs study revealed a high prevalence of ACEs even within a college-educated, middle-class, white majority San Diego population—factors which generally put individuals at less risk for chronic illness.

We applied this approach to a chart review of Bayview children in a primary care setting in 2010–2011 and found that 67 % of children (mean age 8.13) had one or more ACEs and that 12 % had four or more ACEs. Fifty-one percent of the children with four or more ACEs were identified as experiencing learning and behavioral problems. Forty-five percent of those with four or more ACEs were overweight or obese. In comparison, only 3 % of children with zero ACEs experienced learning and behavioral problems, and 31 % were overweight or obese [14]. It became clearer that a response and further prevention was needed to address ACEs in the children from the Bayview community [14].

Introducing the Partners

In order to create an integrated model, different stakeholders needed to come to the table. Representatives from government, academia, community, and philanthropy came together. This founding group consisted of leaders from these various related sectors concerned with addressing child and youth stress and trauma through the lens of each of their fields.

Although we brought together stakeholders from multiple backgrounds, several important voices were missing from the core founders. Educators, for example, who spend such a large amount of time with their students, were not part of the original partnering group. Bringing in teachers and school leaders from the beginning would have informed both how trauma and stress play out in the classroom and highlight the opportunities and limitations present in the public school system to support children and families.

Also missing from the original conversation were members of the police force who may be the first to interface with families and youth in the community. A central actor in addressing violence in the neighborhood, the police department should be included in the conversation as a long-term stakeholder with a strong understanding of the impact of stress and trauma, particularly given the long history of police brutality and resulting distrust among disenfranchised communities in the United States.

Having diverse voices from the community to contribute to the nuanced conversations of implement-

> **Center for Youth Wellness Timeline [15]**
>
> 2007
> Center for Youth Wellness founding partners met to discuss a collaborative approach to early childhood adversity.
>
> SPRING 2010
> Funding partner Tipping Point Community raised more than $4 million for the Center for Youth Wellness building.
>
> SPRING 2012
> Center for Youth Wellness became a 501(c)3 organization.
>
> FALL 2012–SPRING 2013
> Center for Youth Wellness was approved to provide coordinated services in its final location in Bayview Hunters Point.
>
> SPRING 2013
> Center for Youth Wellness began taking referrals from partner organizations and offering clinical services and launched the Community Advisory Council.
>
> WINTER 2014
> Center for Youth Wellness, Bayview Child Health Center, and Children's Advocacy Center opened their doors at the Center for Youth Wellness building.

ing the model in its nascent stages continues to incorporate greater local context and knowledge that is fundamental to maximizing the benefits of such a program for those who will be most impacted by its direction. The Center for Youth Wellness developed community advisory councils and has worked closely with the Bayview Hunters Point neighborhood residents and community-based organizations to inform their decision-making. The organization has collaborated with public schools and offered trainings to the police department as part of their health education programing and wellness coordination. Additionally, the Center for Youth Wellness' research program incorporates community-based participatory research principles to further partner with adult and student stakeholders in the neighborhood.

> *"Having diverse voices from the community to contribute to the nuanced conversations of implementing the model in its nascent stages continues to incorporate greater local context and knowledge that is fundamental to maximizing the benefits of such a program for those who will be most impacted by its direction."*

Our founding group enjoyed a variety of diverse partners working to improve life outcomes in San Francisco, which are described in the following paragraphs.

Tipping Point Community is the Center for Youth Wellness' central funding partner, a grant-making organization focused on alleviating poverty in the Bay Area. Unlike many grant-making organizations, Tipping Point Community offers support such as management and consulting services, real estate or legal support to its nonprofit partners. Tipping Point Community exists to enable the leadership of its grantees, trusting that they can best address a particular problem because their work takes place at the ground level, and giving them the foundational support and resources to focus on their priorities and do their job well.

The University of California, San Francisco's Child Trauma Research Program has been partnering with the Bayview Child Health Center, the primary care seed for the Center for Youth Wellness, providing full-time therapist interns for the past several years. With a focus on dyadic intervention, the Child Trauma Research Program offers child–parent psychotherapy [16] and works to reduce the "mental health gap for underserved communities by providing high-quality training in evidence-based, culturally relevant interventions" for mental health practitioners working with children 5 years old and younger [17].

The San Francisco Child Abuse Prevention Center's Children's Advocacy Center is the primary access, acute services organization for families in crisis. Providing a coordinated first response to child abuse and neglect, the Children's Advocacy Center convenes partners from around the city, including the district attorney's office, the child and victim assault units, child protective services, the police department, and the department of public health. The Children's Advocacy Center is a national model that offers primary forensic, prosecution, mental health, and education services around child abuse and neglect, with a focus on best supporting the family and child through crisis.

Bayview Child Health Center, collocated partner to the Center for Youth Wellness and clinic of California Pacific Medical Center and Sutter Pacific Medical Foundation, is a pediatric clinic that has been open in Bayview since 2007. Offering pediatric, dental, and nutrition services as a primary care organization, the Bayview Child Health Center is the entry point to the center and works to eliminate health disparities in Bayview [18].

The Stanford Early Life Stress and Pediatric Anxiety Program at Lucile Packard Children's Hospital is a founding partner of the Center for Youth Wellness and driver of its clinical research work. With an aim to increase evidence-based interventions from within community-based praxis, the Early Life Stress and Pediatric Anxiety Program now continues to serve as a strategic thought-partner to the Center for Youth Wellness.

The community of Bayview is made up of families and residents, either those who are direct participants—families and their children—in the organization's programming, or residents who, by having lived experiences in the neighborhood, have offered insight and direction for the organization. Community advisory councils exist both for the Center for Youth Wellness' health education and clinical research initiatives and help drive the direction of the organization's programming. They are made up of community leaders and individuals invested in the mission of the Center for Youth Wellness.

Toward an Approach

Because childhood adversity and trauma is such a multifaceted issue and involves stakeholders across disciplines, we saw the need for a wide net of services and support. Chronic stress impacts neurological development, learning and behavior in schools, family and community dynamics, and pediatric and mental health. It is an issue that touches the work of doctors, social workers, educators, parents, policymakers, city planners, academics, and law enforcement, among others. Additionally, due to the sensitive nature and potential for further scapegoating families living in poverty, there is an imperative need to engage families and communities who experience the problem firsthand to become partners and leaders in driving systems-wide change.

In order to develop an integrative model, two organizations in our founding group addressing primary care (the Bayview Child Health Center) and trauma first response and forensic evaluation (the Children's Advocacy Center) collocated with the Center for Youth Wellness in one building known to the community as the Center for Youth Wellness, forming an integrative care structure. We define integrative care here as "the process and product of medical and mental health professionals working collaboratively and coherently toward optimizing patient health through biopsychosocial modes of prevention and intervention" [19]. Each organization relies on one another, utilizing high-quality referrals to connect families to resources "down the hall."

Because both the Children's Advocacy Center and the Center for Youth Wellness were starting out as new organizations, decisions regarding funding, capacity, and operational and programmatic development guided the partnership. With sustainability and capacity in mind, the leadership of both organizations decided to collocate as separate partners along with Bayview Child Health Center. The new direction led to increased flexibility for the partners administratively and operationally, allowing for more focus on carrying out each organization's mission in service of supporting children and families in Bayview.

Another challenge the organizations faced was the timeline, from conception to offering services in Bayview. Conversations among the core group of partners began in 2007, and the centers opened their doors at their final location in early 2014. One of the most pressing challenges during this time was finding a home for the organizations that fit the requirements of each partner and was a safe place for patients and their families. The Center for Youth Wellness began taking referrals from the Bayview Child Health Center when it moved to its temporary location down the street from the health center in early 2013, and offered trainings to educators and other service providers in early 2012.

Partnering

Each partner brought a significant amount of experience and knowledge to the table, contributing to the efficacy of the collocated model of organizations in the Center for Youth Wellness building. Bayview Child Health Center provides general pediatric, dental, and nutrition services to children and youth in Bayview. When children visit for their physical or other pediatric check up, they are screened for ACEs and, if recommended, referred to Center for Youth Wellness staff for further support and therapeutic services. This is done via multidisciplinary rounds, where pediatricians, the wellness coordinator, social workers, nurses, therapists, and case managers meet weekly to discuss patient and family support plans. As part of this model, pediatricians can consult with mental health practitioners about next steps for each family, and families are then consulted to make sure the programming fits their needs.

Within the Children's Advocacy Center, the child is able to tell his or her story, one time, to a licensed and qualified forensic interviewer in a child-friendly atmosphere, and all stakeholders (e.g., police department, child protective services) listen to the story firsthand behind a one-way mirror. Following this first response service, the Children's Advocacy Center offers follow-up support, including case management, acute mental health interventions and services, community education, prosecution, and referrals to the Center for Youth Wellness for long-term programming through the wellness coordinator, a Center for Youth Wellness staff member who coordinates care and acts as an advocate for families across all collaborating organizations.

The Center for Youth Wellness works with families on a longer-term basis, taking referrals from both the Children's Advocacy Center and Bayview Child Health Center. Collaborating also with

> ### Case Study
>
> A 6-year-old patient at Bayview Child Health Center was brought in by his mother for a rash. She also took him to the clinic because he was having behavioral issues at school, where he would often lose control and get in trouble for interrupting, running out of the room, hitting or kicking, and she was concerned.
>
> The boy had experienced a lot of stress, having witnessed domestic violence at home, and a father dealing with addiction who was no longer a part of his life. His now single mother struggled with poverty, trying her best to move forward.
>
> A child going through such stressors has access to several interventions

through the CYW. For example, he might engage in two-generation therapy with his caregiver to address the intergenerational cycle of trauma. This happens by giving the caregiver mental health, social, and logistical resources to support themselves and their children, in addition to providing treatment and support to the child directly. These include interventions like Child-Parent Psychotherapy, mindfulness practices, or other tools.

In this case, the boy received biofeedback, where he was able to watch both how his body reacted to stress and, when he was able to breathe and use other relaxation tools, how his body then calmed down. With the ability to access services such as these, his challenges, several years later, have significantly improved [20].

The Center for Youth wellness coordinator works with patients and their families to access clinical programs and legal, housing, and other resources from service providers in Bayview. Acting as an advocate, the coordinator ensures both initial and ongoing access to these providers and that families have received services.

the University of California San Francisco's Child Trauma Research Program and Stanford's Early Life Stress and Pediatric Anxiety Program's researchers and mental health practitioners, the Center for Youth Wellness provides a variety of evidence-based clinical intervention programs, health education, and training opportunities for other service providers such as local community-based organizations and educators, and leverages their partners' cohesive effort to impact policy at the state and national level around childhood trauma and pediatric practice.

Now offering full services, the Center for Youth Wellness model works through several branches that continue to evolve: treatment and practice, research and evaluation, and education and advocacy.

Center for Youth Wellness Structure and Programs

The Center for Youth Wellness is made up of a founding board from various stakeholder organizations and has a leadership team of chief and vice president roles. A cohort of directors leads each focus of the organization and its sub-teams: research, clinical program, development, strategic initiatives, and organizational learning and data. Community advisory councils guide the direction of organizational practice in Center for Youth Wellness research and community programs.

Working in a new health center following the trauma-informed system of care structure, Center for Youth Wellness staff share a number of traditions and values. First, each staff member, regardless of his or her role, receives training on trauma and chronic stress in order to better support patients throughout the center. Another large part of this model is staff wellness; therefore, not only is mutual respect and support across teams integral but also are opportunities for staff to care for themselves as individuals. For example, weekly staff meetings begin with shout-outs, where staff members call out someone else for their hard work, something positive they had done that week, or an accomplishment. Each meeting ends with a couple of minutes of silent meditation before moving on with the rest of the day.

Treatment and Practice

In partnership with Bayview Child Health Center, patients receive pediatric, dental, and nutrition services with their primary care provider. During these routine visits, all children and youth are screened for exposure to ACEs and, on the basis of their score, are referred for a variety of wellness services through the Center for Youth Wellness. Clinical interventions at the Center for Youth Wellness are trauma-focused and incorporate a two-generation approach; caregivers are heavily involved with Center for Youth Wellness services so they can best support their children in their healing.

Evidence-based intervention therapies include trauma-focused cognitive-behavioral therapy, child–parent psychotherapy, and Stanford's cue-centered therapy. Mindfulness meditation, yoga, and biofeedback are part of the Center for Youth Wellness' clinical interventions. Family needs can also be identified via home visits, conducted by the wellness coordinator, a Center for Youth Wellness staff member. The wellness coordinator works across the three partnering organizations to be an advocate for the family and not only secure the biomedical and mental health needs of family members but also identify them and connect the family members to other resources such as legal, housing, food, or other assistance. In addition, understanding the significant benefits of nutrition and exercise, the Center for Youth Wellness is currently develop-

---

Community-Based Participatory Research and the Legacy of Henrietta Lacks

The case of Henrietta Lacks [21], an African American woman who died of cervical cancer in the 1950s and whose cervical cells were taken without her permission or knowledge, is now well known. Her cells have contributed to both a legacy of medical advances and an important discussion about ethics and power regarding the history of research in low-income communities and communities of color, among other groups historically disenfranchised in the US.

The rights and empowerment of communities involved in research are still an issue today. Community-based participatory research is one tool to help mitigate the negative impact health research can have on its "subjects" by engaging them as full participants and leaders in the research process.

As part of the Center for Youth Wellness' research initiative, Henrietta Lacks' family was invited to Bayview to meet with residents in October 2014. Questions around trust, community participation in research, and bias in the scientific community, among others, were discussed.

This meeting is an example of how the Center for Youth Wellness research program works with community members to create knowledge and systemic change around negative health outcomes.

---

ing programs in these areas. The wellness coordinator both refers families to these services and follows up to make sure the family is able to access and utilize them.

Research and Evaluation

The research and evaluation team at the Center for Youth Wellness works with practitioners and researchers from Stanford's Early Life Stress and Pediatric Anxiety Program that initially drove the research arm of the organization through years of research around stress, brain function, and development. Working to increase evidenced-based therapies in community mental health, the research team also functions to evaluate the entire model of the Center for Youth Wellness on the basis of patient outcomes after receiving clinical services. In order to conduct research that is culturally respectful and sustainable, the research team is developing a community-based research advisory board and is utilizing a community-based participatory research orientation as part of the program. Leveraging these principles, the research program engages community members and students in critical research projects.

Education and Advocacy

The Center for Youth Wellness staff and board members work as advocates by disseminating information on the impact of ACEs and toxic stress on children, both at the state and national level, and by supporting other service providers around California. The chief executive officer of the Center for Youth Wellness, for example, serves as part of Hillary Rodham Clinton's Too Small to Fail Campaign, the Let's Get Healthy California task force, and the American Association of Pediatrics. The scientific advisory board chairman is a member of the Mental Health Oversight and Accountability Commission for California and the American Association of Child and Adolescent Psychiatry.

Utilizing curricula developed with Stanford partners based on clinical praxis, Center for Youth Wellness staff train other public sector organizations on trauma and ACEs, including public school educators and pediatricians. In particular, the Center for Youth Wellness is working as a technical assistance provider to the Positive Youth Justice Initiative, which aims to "support juvenile justice system redesign at the county level to produce better outcomes for crossover youth" [22]. Given its work on the ground with the support of experts in various aspects of ACEs and toxic stress, the Center for Youth Wellness is uniquely positioned to inform local, state, and national policies.

Additionally, the Center for Youth Wellness works with other organizations that have been offering services in Bayview, including Hunters Point Family, BMagic, and public schools in the neighborhood. Relying on high-quality referrals, the Center for Youth Wellness depends consistently on its partner organizations within the community to connect families to the resources they need, such as housing, legal, and financial services. The Center for Youth Wellness also works with these community-based organizations to provide programming around trauma and wellness. Hunters Point Family, for example, who has partnered with the Center for Youth Wellness to provide programming for youth and their parents, is a grass-roots organization that has been in Bayview since 1997. The organization offers various educational, leadership, and professional resources to youth in the neighborhood.

Considerations and Lessons Learned

We identified three areas that were centrally important to staff members and Center for Youth Wellness stakeholders: (1) transparency and authenticity, (2) celebrating partner work, and (3) a clear understanding of one's limitations and capacity and clarity around each stakeholder's role with a strong understanding of and focus on shared goals.

Stakeholders felt it was imperative for all partners to come to the table with authenticity about who they are as individuals and why they do this work. Part of this authenticity is the ability to be transparent about decision-making rationale, values, and motives, with the understanding that this transparency builds trust among partners while allowing for different perspectives. For example, the ability of practitioners not only to recognize their relative privilege but also to understand how it impacts their role in the community and to act upon that understanding has great potential to benefit the work long-term.

Valuing partners was also a central aspect of building the model. This meant not only engaging members of the community but also respecting the knowledge and perspective that each partner brings. In this vein, partners need to truly listen to one another and meet each other where they are, whether that is toward a family who is not yet ready to engage in therapy or another service provider who has similar values and a different approach. Specifically for residents of Bayview and families who may experience the chronic stress and trauma of poverty firsthand, this

> **Center for Youth Wellness Model**
>
> 1. Collocation of holistic pediatric and mental health services to address health outcomes using Adverse Childhood Experiences (ACEs) as a diagnostic tool.
> 2. Wellness coordinator role to act as family advocate and coordinate CYW and other service provider programs and resources.
> 3. Research program focused on evidence-based praxis and engaging community members to conduct research on health outcomes in Bayview.
> 4. Education program that works to increase the capacity of other service providers around chronic stress and trauma.
> 5. Policy and advocacy initiatives at the local, state, and national level grounded in evidence-based praxis and research.

meant actively recruiting from the neighborhood for staff positions.

> *"…there is an appreciation, again, of what their partners bring to the table and understanding that one organization cannot "do it all." This is not only important for a successful partnership, but for sustainability as a service provider."*

Additionally, working in a startup
environment through a model that heavily
relies on interdependent functioning and
strategic partnership proved to be difficult
in some ways, particularly for clarity
around scope and responsibility of individual roles. Staff felt that the flexibility
in their roles was important, as their work streams might shift in the iterative process of
developing the organization, but noted that in a partnership it is helpful to know who
owns what, so that expectations are aligned. For the wellness coordinator this is especially important as he or she, although a Center for Youth Wellness staff member, coordinates services for families between both the collocated organizations at the Center and
other service providers in the neighborhood. Additionally, for example, a physician at
Bayview Child Health Center would need to understand the role of a Center for Youth
Wellness mental health provider in order to make the appropriate referral for a patient.
Part of what makes this doable is for each stakeholder to have clear knowledge of his or
her focus and capacity, either as an individual or an organization; this way there is an
appreciation, again, of what their partners bring to the table and understanding that one
organization cannot "do it all." This is not only important for a successful partnership
but also for sustainability as a service provider.

Future Directions

Although the Center for Youth Wellness, the Children's Advocacy Center, and the
Bayview Child Health Center only opened their doors as a cohesive unit in the
beginning of 2014, staff and other stakeholders have already identified considerations for other practitioners interested in building a similar model in the future.

For those looking to start a similar model in another area of the United States, the
importance of combining pediatric and mental health services, research, and policy
is what led to the Center for Youth Wellness' identity. Each of these parts, along with
high-quality referral practices, contributes to what makes the Center for Youth
Wellness an evidence-based, holistic model of health care. Practitioners wanting to
collocate with a child advocacy center will find that many exist across the United
States; however, the models vary by local context and child advocacy centers may
already be partnering with other organizations.

Practitioners should follow the model in order to avoid recreating the wheel
unnecessarily. And although the core model is important, it is essential to know the
community and its history, understand who they are and what their needs are, and
involve them in the process. Respect for stakeholder perspectives is central, whether
for patient families and local residents or for community-based organizations who
have been doing work in the community for some time. Ultimately, having respect

for and understanding community needs may alter the model, but if practitioners remember to start small, this should be manageable.

This partnership model is part of an ongoing and iterative process of learning. As the organization conducts more research on the model and receives feedback from stakeholders, it will continue to evolve. The core facets of community, academic, government, medical, and other public sector partnerships, however, remain integral to its potential as a holistic, trauma-informed, and community-based model of health care and wellness.

References

1. Shonkoff JP, Garner AS, Committee on Psychosocial Aspects of Child and Family Health, Committee on Early Childhood, Adoption, and Dependent Care, Section on Developmental and Behavioral Pediatrics. The lifelong effects of early childhood adversity and toxic stress. Pediatrics. 2012;129:e232–46.
2. Centers for Disease Control and Prevention. Web-based injury statistics query and reporting system. Atlanta, GA: Centers for Disease Control and Prevention. Available at http://www.cdc.gov/injury/wisqars/. Last accessed 9 Mar 2014.
3. National Association of Community Health Centers. Community health center funding declines as demand for services rises. Bethesda, MD: National Association of Community Health Centers. Available at http://www.nachc.com/magazine-article.cfm?MagazineArticle ID=201. Last accessed 7 Mar 2014.
4. Campbell PH, Halbert J. Between research and practice: provider perspectives on early intervention. Topics Early Child Spec Educ. 2002;22:211–24.
5. Weisz JR, Weersing VR. Psychotherapy with children and adolescents: efficacy, effectiveness and developmental concerns. In: Cicchetti D, Toth SL, editors. Rochester symposium on developmental psychopathology, Developmental approaches to prevention and intervention, vol. 9. Rochester, NY: University of Rochester Press; 1999. p. 341–86.
6. Corburn J. Confronting the challenges in reconnecting urban planning and public health. Am J Public Health. 2004;94:541–6.
7. Katz MH. Health programs in Bayview Hunter's Point and recommendations for improving the health of Bayview Hunter's Point Residents. San Francisco, CA: San Francisco Department of Public Health, Office of Policy and Planning; 2006.
8. San Francisco Burden of Disease and Injury Study: Determinants of Health. San Francisco, CA: Department of Public Health. Available at http://www.healthysf.org/bdi/outcomes/94124. Last accessed 7 Mar 2014.
9. Gottlieb L, Sandel M, Adler N. Collecting and applying data on social determinants of health in health care settings. JAMA Intern Med. 2013;173:1017–20.
10. Department of Health and Human Services, Centers for Medicare and Medicaid Services. Federally qualified health center. Baltimore, MD: Centers for Medicare and Medicaid Services. Available at https://www.cms.gov/Outreach-and-Education/Medicare-Learning-Network-MLN/MLNProducts/downloads/fqhcfactsheet.pdf. Last accessed 23 Mar 2014.
11. Minnesota Association of Community Health Centers. Is FQHC a fit for your community? 2014. Available at http://www.mnachc.org/fqhc.html. Last accessed 22 Mar 2014.
12. Prentice B. Bay Area Regional Health Inequities Initiative. Health inequities in the Bay Area. Bay Area, CA: Public Health Institute, Bay Area Regional Health Inequities Initiative; 2008.
13. Felitti VJ, Anda RF, Nordenberg D, Williamson DF, Spitz AM, Edwards V, et al. Relationship of childhood abuse and household dysfunction to many of the leading causes of death in adults: the Adverse Childhood Experiences (ACE) Study. Am J Prev Med. 1998;14:245–58.

14. Burke NJ, Hellman JL, Scott BG, Weems CF, Carrion VG. The impact of adverse childhood experiences on an urban pediatric population. Child Abuse Negl. 2011;35:408–13.
15. Center for Youth Wellness. Our Story. Available at http://centerforyouthwellness.org/about/our-story/. Last accessed 4 Nov 2014; and http://centerforyouthwellness.org/blog/Lacks.
16. Lieberman AF, Ghosh Ippen C, Van Horn P. Child-parent psychotherapy: 6-month follow-up of a randomized controlled trial. J Am Acad Child Adolesc Psychiatry. 2006;45:913–8.
17. University of California, San Francisco. Child Trauma Research Program. Available at http://childtrauma.ucsf.edu/. Last accessed 9 Mar 2014.
18. Sutter Health California Pacific Medical Center. Available at http://www.cpmc.org/. Last accessed 9 Mar 2014.
19. O'Donahue W, Henderson DA, Byrd M, Cummings NA. Behavioral integrative care: treatments that work in primary care setting. New York: Brunner-Routledge; 2005.
20. Burke Harris N. The chronic stress of poverty: toxic to children. Available from: http://shriverreport.org/the-chronic-stress-of-poverty-toxic-to-children-nadine-burke-harris/. Last accessed 2 Nov 2014.
21. Skloot R. The immortal life of Henrietta lacks. New York: Random House, Inc.; 2010.
22. Sierra Health Foundation. Positive Youth Justice Initiative. Available at https://www.sierrahealth.org/assets/PYJI_Briefing_Paper_Reprint_2013.pdf. Last accessed 22 Mar 2014.

Narrative 4

The Cambodian Lotus Thrives Under a California Sun: How a Mental Health Clinic Partnered with a Khmer Buddhist Temple to Reach Killing Fields Refugees Living in California

Daryn Reicherter, Sophany Bay, Bophal Phen, Tith Chan, and Yeon Soo Lee

This is a story borne out of crisis—the collaboration between a mental health clinic and a Khmer Buddhist temple to provide care for community residents, including refugees of the Killing Fields living in California.

D. Reicherter, M.D. (✉)
Department of Psychiatry and Behavioral Sciences, Stanford University School of Medicine, Stanford, CA, USA
e-mail: reichertermd@yahoo.com

S. Bay, M.H.R.S
Gardner Family Care Corporation, Cambodian Program, San Jose, CA, USA
e-mail: sbay@gfc-corp.org

B. Phen, M.H.T., L.C.S.W
Gardner Family Care Corporation, Cambodian Program, San Jose, CA, USA
e-mail: bphen@gfc-corp.org

T. Chan, M.H.T., A.S.W.
Gardner Family Care Corporation, Cambodian Program, San Jose, CA 95112, USA
e-mail: tchan@gfc-corp.org

Y.S. Lee, M.H.T, L.C.S.W
Gardner Family Care Corporation, APYP/Cambodian Program, San Jose, CA, USA
e-mail: ylee@gfc-corp.org

© Springer International Publishing Switzerland 2015
L.W. Roberts et al. (eds.), *Partnerships for Mental Health*,
DOI 10.1007/978-3-319-18884-3_4

The Story of Sophany Bay, Mental Health Specialist

I am a survivor of the Khmer Rouge, Pol Pot regime. Almost 4 years in that cruel regime, I had experiences in life which was so sad, so painful, and plentiful of sufferings that I carry until now. I lost my three children, my whole family to the regime because of killings, starvation, and sickness. I lived with fear, daily, and waited for the end of my life by the Khmer Rouge soldiers. Almost 40 years ago. Nightmares and bad dreams still occur and I still scream at night and wake up my husband who sleep near me. He wonders why I still have nightmares, and it is because all pictures of my children, my parents, my siblings, and family still stick in my memory.

The terrific events! The killings of people in front of my face! I lived in a dark place that the rest of the world did not understand and did not see me and see the Cambodian people in that time. The past trauma still bothers me today. My life in the United States with my husband makes me find peace and a safe place to live, but the nightmare still haunts me.

A proverb says that life is a struggle. The French say, *La vie c'est une lutte.* This proverb encourages me to be strong, to struggle for life if I want to live to see the world, the world of justice. I have to be strong to survive and to face any difficulties of life without my children, my parents and my siblings and my family anymore. They are all gone. My new life is with my handicapped husband who was paralyzed from stroke, depression, lack of hope, helplessness, and stress.

I was a schoolteacher before in my country, Cambodia. Why do I have to step down to destroy my life, to ruin my life as an educated person? I have to struggle for life as the proverb said. So, by thinking about that I try to survive to build up my strength and to motivate myself, to maintain my daily life functioning with my poor husband.

I became a Cambodian mental health counselor from 1988 helping my people who have the same problem as me to live with peace and without fear and to reduce symptoms of PTSD that they carried with them for many years, and to reduce depression from different kinds of things they faced.

I am a Buddhist. That is my national religion that my family practiced so long from generation to generation. I am able to use Buddhist philosophy to handle my job as counselor and help my people to be like me. I believe they trust me in healing their wounds that they carry for so many years. Believing in Buddha makes survivors and people find peace, having less depression, less stress, and less worries by practicing meditation, and mindfulness. Along with medication from our psychiatrist, they feel better, and the symptoms of posttraumatic stress disorder and depression decrease. Our psychiatrist believes that too. That's why Gardner mental health agency opened meditation classes years ago for clients by inviting the monk to come to present in the class and provide knowledge of mindfulness. I'm a facilitator of the class. With the practice of meditation and medication from psychiatrist, Cambodian patients become less depressed, less anxious, less thinking, and less stress. They are getting better and better like the lotus flowers growing in the Cambodian community in the United States.

From "Day Zero" to Freedom

The lotus is a powerful symbol in Khmer Buddhism. It grows out of murky water to bloom into a pure and beautiful flower, just as the mind grows out of chaos into enlightenment in Khmer Buddhist philosophy. Lotus blossoms abound in the wetlands of Cambodia. This beautiful symbol was witness to one of the most brutal mass crimes in recent history.

On April 17, 1975, Pol Pot declared "day zero." He executed a nefarious military plan with bizarre and cruel social-political goals. Pol Pot's reign of terror and genocide dismantled the social structure of a kingdom. More than a million people were murdered in "the Killing Fields" of Cambodia. Their nameless graves are peppered with wild Cambodian lotus.

In the aftermath of the Khmer Rouge, hundreds of thousands of traumatized refugees fled into neighboring countries with stories of incredible violence, torture, starvation, and witnessed murder. Pol Pot's killing machine targeted for execution the educated, the politically connected, the brokers of culture or art. The poor and illiterate agricultural population was spared murder but was terrorized, tortured, starved, and raped. And upon escape from the Khmer Rouge's grasp, the survivors' only hope was to scramble through the lotus fields and into Thailand [1].

Over the decade that followed, more than 150,000 terrorized refugees were resettled to the United States. Many illiterate and monolingual, most traumatized, Khmer survivors were disseminated to host cities from California to Massachusetts. Prevalence of trauma-related mental health disorders was beyond rates seen in almost any other sample population [2].

San Jose, California, received 10,000 Cambodian refugees. There were no culturally competent mental health resources in the city.

In the shadow of the Silicon Valley Tech industry, a Cambodian lotus was planted in the garden of a new Buddhist temple.

No one knew whether it would grow there.

The Story of Bophal Phen, Social Worker

I was born and raised in Cambodia. Growing up, I was repeatedly exposed to life-and-death situations and forced to go on survival mode. By age 10, I had lived through a devastating civil war, and by age 14, I had survived a horrible genocide. I was deprived of an opportunity to attend school and enjoy life without fear, danger, and violence. So when the war was over, I felt ecstatic and heavenly, jumping up and down, running around smiling and laughing, and playing outside like a carefree preadolescent. At last, there was peace, and there was no more fear. There were no more bombs dropping from the sky, destroying lives, villages, and properties. There were no more explosions in crowded places, injuring and killing innocent people.

But peace was short-lived, and my heaven turned into hell in a matter of days.

In 1975, the Cambodian communist guerrillas, commonly known as the Khmer Rouge, took complete control over the country. Dressed in black and armed with guns, the Khmer Rouge soldiers went around the cities telling people to flee to the countryside. They said, "The Americans are coming to drop bombs on us." Heeding their warning, my family and I headed to the countryside with very few belongings, hoping to return home within 3 days. Once in the countryside, however, we along with thousands of other evacuees were not allowed to return to the cities. Instead, we were forcibly assigned to different rural villages and told to follow Angkar's directives without questions. For those who resisted, the punishment was death. The Khmer Rouge's motto was "To keep you is no gain, and to kill you is no loss." My family and I were eventually relocated several times, and each time our lives became more and more miserable.

During the Khmer Rouge's reign of terror, which lasted for almost 4 years, I was separated from my parents and four siblings. My father, two older brothers, and an older sister were assigned to different mobile units, and they were sent to work in the rice fields. My younger brother and I were initially allowed to stay with our mother, but later on, I was placed in a makeshift shelter for teens. We were forced to work in the rice fields from dawn to dusk, weeding and clearing plots of land, building dams and dikes, digging canals, transporting and transplanting rice seedlings, and gleaning the fields after harvest time. Day in and day out, I had to work under very harsh conditions and was given two meals of rice porridge to eat for lunch and dinner. I was starved and wasted away and had to eat anything that I could get my hands on, like roots, aquatic plants, fruits, honeycombs, rats, fish, frogs, birds, and insects. I was caught for stealing and while foraging for food many times, and these "immoral" transgressions were punishable by death for adults. But I was young, and so the Khmer Rouge cadres were more lenient with me. They arrested me, tied my hands behind my back, detained me, and threatened to kill me. I was "re-educated" for putting my self-interest before that of Angkar. I saw many people disappearing and dying and knew what had happened to them. The majority of them were executed while the rest died from overwork, starvation, and diseases. The Khmer Rouge cadres banned almost everything and strictly enforced the directives of Angkar. They were the enforcers, the judges, and the executioners. I was on my own and had to do my best to survive. I got really sick on two separate occasions, and each time I almost died. My parents and siblings were sent to different locations, and we hardly saw each other for almost 4 years. Fortunately, our family was reunited in 1979 when the Vietnamese armies invaded Cambodia and toppled the Khmer Rouge regime. After the civil war and genocide, I lost one older brother, two older sisters, and one younger sister to ailments and execution. My parents had ten children in total, and these four had been either deceased or displaced from the family.

The 1979 invasion and occupation of Cambodia by the Vietnamese armed forces caused a massive exodus of Cambodian refugees. Thousands of these Killing Fields survivors escaped to the Thai-Cambodian border. My parents had second thoughts about staying put, and they were afraid of being persecuted by the Vietnamese. As a result, we decided to flee with others, despite knowing how dangerous the trek was.

The danger was everywhere, from landmines, Vietnamese soldiers, Thai soldiers, Khmer Rouge soldiers, resistance soldiers, and armed robbers. My family and I ended up living in refugee camps for years, and we were subjected to indescribable horror and misery. But while staying in these refugee camps and waiting for outside help, I finally had an opportunity to go to school. In 1983, my family and I were allowed to resettle in America. By this time, I had lived through years of civil war, survived the genocidal communist regime, and endured innumerable hardships while migrating. Through these adversities, I had learned to survive under harsh conditions and to appreciate the support from family. Also, I had learned to be strong, persistent, and optimistic, and as it turned out, these qualities served me well in my new world. I was able to deal with difficulties and challenges while getting adjusted to my new life and transitioning to early adulthood.

Survivors in a New Land

The survivors had experienced unspeakable conditions and suffered beyond imagination. Their resettlement in the United States became a major challenge for the Office of Resettlement and for the host cities throughout the states that accepted the immigration. The mental health issues were overwhelming. And this wave of refugees had undergone selection forces for poor acculturation through the nature of Pol Pot's killing machine. Many were poor, illiterate, monolingual, agricultural persons without experience of modern technology. Most were victims of grave human rights abuses.

Poor Access to Mental Health Care

Survivors were relocated to host cities throughout the United States. Many individuals with horror stories found themselves in a strange new reality without language capacity, without financial resources, and entirely unprepared for acculturation. Given the overwhelming mental health burden, most resettled Cambodian groups had great disadvantage even accessing the social welfare or health care system in their new cities. San Jose, California, was no exception. The Khmer population quickly found itself at the low end of the socioeconomic scale, without access to basic needs. Cambodians in San Jose did not seek mental health treatment because they did not understand their condition to be in the category of "mental health." Furthermore, if they did want health care, they did not feel that they had access. Most had no medical coverage or Medicaid at best. And most did not know how to use it if they had it [3]. The Khmer community had limited health care resources, each other, and a local Buddhist temple.

Illustration: "Incomplete Execution"[1]

S.Y. was a poor street merchant in Cambodia when the Pol Pot regime took power. He witnessed the total destruction of the social fabric of his society. He witnessed the forced evacuation of Phnom Pen and the murder/execution of civilians who did not follow the orders of soldiers. They were executed before his eyes with guns, beatings, and beheadings. He was forced to watch the execution of family members, and he was separated from his children. He was placed into a work camp, where he underwent torture and hard labor in the context of starvation.

He was slotted for execution when his commander decided he was an "enemy of the communist party." He was lined up for mass execution with other citizens in front of "the killing fields." The executioner used a garden hoe to chop the back of the neck of his victims. He was among the last in a line of about 50 kneeling victims, and somehow the executioner's hoe only blasted the back of his head, not murdering him. His unconscious body was hurled into a mass grave with the rotting corpses of a thousand countrymen. But he was not dead. Blinded by the blow and bleeding, he awoke in the field under a shallow grave of bodies and dirt. He escaped, feeling his way across the killing fields and into the jungle. He would certainly have been executed at any moment had he encountered a Khmer Rouge soldier. Partially blind and starving, he was able to negotiate his way through the Cambodian jungle. He staggered through the forest mostly by night for months until he reached the Thai border.

He never saw his wife or children again.

He was evacuated to the US as a refugee 5 years after he escaped from Cambodia.

He was relocated to the low-income area of San Jose, California. He suffered with severe symptoms of posttraumatic stress disorder. He dreaded sleeping because his nightmares would pull him back to his shallow grave, next to the stinking bodies he had lain with. He did not have a concept of his condition as a "mental health disorder." Rather, he thought, "I was going crazy. I was insane." He did not have access to a culturally, linguistically competent provider to help him. He hid in his small apartment, haunted by the shadows of his past. He had no resource for mental health.

---

[1] This case illustration represents the narratives of several patients and is typical of individuals in the clinic.

Where To Go for Partnership

San Jose and Santa Clara County Mental Health acknowledged an enormous gap between the mental health need and delivery of services for this population by creating special funding for a Cambodian Family Mental Health Program. Our clinic answered the call. Gardner Family Care Corporation is a nonprofit mental health clinic in San Jose, California, that serves vulnerable populations and specializes in culturally informed care. We established a team of Khmer cultural experts with language and culture capacity. Moreover, we created a team of professionals with the right *experience* to heal this population. Some of their personal and professional stories told in this narrative give a sense of how interwoven their experience is with that of the intended community we intended to serve.

The story of partnership to address this major health care disparity starts with the joining of persons with a common mission. A California-born psychiatrist and a team of Cambodian-born Khmer Americans joined together. The coauthors of this narrative include Khmer survivors turned healers. Their personal stories are inspirational and compelling and are the root of their essential ingredient to the partnership. But the need for another element of reaching the broader Khmer community brought us a new partner.

The Most Unusual Partner

Getting started took multiple inputs. We used the experience of our Khmer clinicians as well as the professional expertise of a Western-trained psychiatrist. But without the mix, the *lotus* would never have bloomed. And without another partner, we could not reach the population we hoped to serve. The community partner needed to complete the program was not a health care provider at all.

A mental health clinic is definitely not the center of Khmer community life. In fact, there is huge stigma against mental illness. The Khmer community is centered on the Buddhist temple. The great majority of Cambodians are Buddhist. Cambodia's major provider of spiritual and community needs is the Buddhist temple. And the monks take the role of community organizers and advocates as well as spiritual leaders. In order to achieve true buy-in for the community's utility of mental health services, we needed to partner with the leaders of the community. In doing so, we achieved much more than we initially had hoped.

The Story of Daryn Reicherter, Psychiatrist

I spent a month in Cambodia as a psychiatrist learning about how trauma-related mental health is dealt with there. (I would later go on to visit and consult there over the next many years.) "Mental health" wasn't the same thing there. Trauma psychology was extremely prevalent, but the symptoms of posttraumatic stress disorder were not seen as an issue for a health care provider. Most Cambodians with PTSD symptoms went to the local Buddhist temples to seek a cure. I met with monks and abbots in Cambodia to learn about what they do with the symptoms I call PTSD. They described a community approach to trauma-related mental health issues. They open the temple as a community resource center. And they use Buddhist meditation as a remedy for symptoms of anxiety.

Great solution, I thought, if only my clinic in San Jose had access to a temple.

When I returned from Cambodia to my clinic, I had many new ideas for clinical outcomes research for my Khmer mental health patients. I wanted to implement a similar paradigm for the Khmer patients in my clinic and do community-based research on the outcomes. But to incorporate such a function, our community-based clinic would need a Khmer Buddhist monk. Initially I thought this would be a tall order in California relative to Cambodia.

Sophany said, "Why don't you just go and meet the monks in San Jose?" I didn't know there was one. But she was an active member of the Khmer community and knew the abbot of the local temple, a Khmer Krom Buddhist monk and human rights advocate.

After Sophany's introduction, the monk invited me to join him for a "Dharma talk at the next new moon." I waited until the new moon and then went to the temple that day. The monk taught me some basic principles of Buddhist thought, and we sat together in quite meditation. When we finished, he stood up and excused himself.

He invited me to come to the temple on a weekly basis, each time offering a Dharma lecture and a meditation experience. Initially, he did not want to talk about partnership; rather, he wanted to teach me this method of meditation. I went week after week.

We met. He taught. We meditated. I learned.

This went on for one lunar cycle before the subject of formal partnership came up again. He had used the regular meetings for two purposes. He needed to establish a trust with me to satisfy his concern over whether I was dedicated to our common service population. He was interested in working with me and with our clinic but needed to make sure that my commitment was true and that the work, in the end, would be for the benefit of the Khmer community. Also, he wanted me to know the method and the process of the meditations in an experiential way before I was to incorporate them into a solution for survivors.

We met separately from the meditation sessions to develop the partnership plan. We met at the clinic to formalize the partnership and met at the temple to continue learning meditation. This feature of partnering with the temple was important because we were acknowledging the difference between a sacred place (the temple) and a business place (the clinic).

Meditation groups were designed specifically to use basic Khmer Buddhist techniques for the cessation of anxiety symptoms. The temple began hosting meditation groups and also providing meditation groups at our clinic. The monks began co-leading meditation sessions with Khmer mental health specialists for survivors. Patients used the sessions held at the clinic. The temple hosted sessions for the community (patients and non-patients).

I was welcomed to join the abbot for weekly meditation with the other monks in a separate meditation. I participated in silent meditation with the monks at the temple for 3 years.

Partnership

Our clinic became partners with the temple Wat Khmara Rangsey through the influence of the Khmer clinicians and a slow, mutually respectful dialogue focused on the needs of the shared target population. Both the temple and the clinic had the needs of the Khmer community in mind, but true dialogue was necessary to determine a partnership approach that would work best. The dialogue had to be very honest and very understanding in order to work. Two very different philosophies had to be reconciled.

Neither group was pushing its own worldview. Rather, each group was open to the other's ideas. We discussed solutions. We agreed. Sometimes, we did not see things the same way. But we were able to listen to each other and come up with compromises (or even change mindsets).

Listening is the most fertile ground for the ground of a partnership.

> *"Both the temple and the clinic had the needs of the Khmer community in mind, but true dialogue was necessary to determine a partnership approach that would work best. The dialogue had to be very honest and very understanding in order to work. Two very different philosophies had to be reconciled."*

Wat Khmara Rangsey

The temple Wat Khmara Rangsey became a wellness outreach site for our clinic. Our providers began to run a wellness program at the temple.

The clinic became a wellness outreach site for the temple. The monks became volunteers at the clinic and ran culturally sensitive wellness functions alongside our providers.

Meditation Groups

The partnership between the temple and the clinic became a key in reaching the Khmer community.

Although the meditation groups became an intrinsic part of the behavioral intervention for our mental health program in the clinic, the other aspects of partnership were invaluable as well. The design for this intervention was very simple and entirely consistent with Western models of behavioral, relaxation techniques.

The Khmer clinicians worked with the monks to tailor Buddhist meditation themes into behavioral interventions specifically targeting symptoms of PTSD. This discourse occurred over a reasonably short time course because the basic program of the monks' teaching lent to behavioral psychiatry. The program was formalized as a synthesis of behavioral psychology techniques and millennia-old Buddhist methods. It occurs in weekly, 2-hour sessions, for a 12-week period. Groups are taught by ordained monks in the Khmer language and co-led by licensed mental health staff. Patients relate very well to the "class" as a social, spiritual, and therapeutic function [4].

The Story of Bophal Penh, Social Worker (Continued)

I was enrolled in high school at the age of 18 and able to graduate within 3 years. Throughout these years, my family and I were on welfare, and the entire family became increasingly chaotic and dysfunctional. My parents' health, both physical and mental, was deteriorating due to old age, alcohol and tobacco abuse, past traumatic experiences, and acculturation stress. My mother had multiple health conditions that required frequent medical attention and hospitalizations. My father suffered from chronic obstructive pulmonary disease and congestive heart failure and required frequent medical treatments and hospitalizations. I became their caretaker while attending college. In 1998, I graduated with a baccalaureate degree in psychology.

A year later, I got a job at Gardner Family Care Corporation, working as a mental health rehabilitation specialist. I provided culturally competent services to non-English-speaking and traumatized Cambodian clients. I also co-facilitated youth group, meditation group, men's group, and parents' group. While working, volunteering, and taking care of my ailing parents, I attended graduate school and graduated in 2010 with a master's degree in social work. Two years later, I became a licensed clinical social worker. I now continue to work with mostly Cambodian adults, rehabilitating them, helping them with life skills, and linking them to other specialists and community resources.

Special Issues in Cross-Cultural, Khmer-Specific Work

Although there are general realities of trauma-related mental health outcomes that seem to be applicable across cultural experience, the nuances of culture-specific presentations of psychological experience must not be ignored. One description of post-traumatic stress disorder outlines the general syndrome of symptom constellation that can occur after terrible trauma [5]. But it does not prepare providers for the particulars of trauma psychology in a cultural context. This is certainly true in the Khmer "killing fields" survivors with subsequent trauma-related mental health symptoms. So many nuances are present in Khmer presentations of PTSD that faculty at Harvard created a Khmer-specific addendum to the standard PTSD checklist [6].

For those practitioners ignorant to cultural presentations of mental health disorders, the Khmer presentation of PTSD and other trauma-related mental health issues might not be obvious. Clinicians could misinterpret common cultural idioms of distress as psychotic pathology. Without the discourse with a cultural expert, inaccurate diagnoses and inappropriate treatment plans can be enacted [7].

Our cultural expertise with our clinic's cultural expert providers and our partnership with the temple have helped clarify the diagnosis and treatment of patients and also helped to educate the community toward mental health issues. They have broken down the stigma related to mental health symptoms and allowed for improved access to treatment.

Outcomes

The partnership with the Khmer temple is invaluable for our target population. It has rounded out the cross-cultural capacity of the clinic to the extent that the community trusts and uses the clinical services without the usual biases associated with stigma. In fact, the clinic will receive "referrals" from the monks for community members that they recognize as suffering with anxiety or other mental health symptoms. The clinic also "refers" patients to the temple for psycho-education groups, social services, and social events.

We all spend Khmer New Year together.

Cambodian Culturally-Specific Family Services (CCFC) of Gardner Family Care Corporation has been proving culturally and linguistically competent mental health services for Cambodian children, adults, and families in Santa Clara County since 1999. CCFC services include individual therapy, group therapy or counseling, rehabilitation, case management, medication support, and crisis intervention. The services are provided in a variety of settings, such as clinics, home, school, and other locations in the community, and the services are culturally tailored for those who are not familiar with Western culture. Annually, the average of 80–90 adult, child, and older adult clients have been receiving services to improve their life functioning.

CCFC has developed and implemented a culturally competent group counseling named as mindfulness meditation group with the collaboration with United Khmer Temple in 2006. The meditation group was designed to be facilitated by a Mental Health Rehabilitation Specialist and a Buddhist monk, focusing on meditation practice and lesson with discussion of Buddhism concepts. The first meditation group consisted of six sessions and started in October 2006 with participation of nine clients, followed by another meditation group of seven sessions in March 2007. As of August 2007, the meditation group formed as a regular program with 12 sessions consisting of introduction and Buddhist concepts such as metta, karuna, mudita, upekkha, and purification. Each topic was discussed for 2 weeks with meditation practice, and the topic of the previous session was reviewed in the beginning of each session in order to enhance cumulative learning and life application.

An evaluation was conducted for the effectiveness of the mindfulness group utilizing one group pre/post-test design during Fall 2007. A total of 9 Cambodian adult clients among 57 clients who have symptoms of PTSD participated in the 12 sessions of mindfulness meditation and the evaluation study, and the severity of PTSD symptoms was measured before the participants attended the group and after they completed the 12 sessions. The results showed that all participants reported markedly reduced PTSD after the mindfulness meditation group [8].

After the study, CCFC continued mindfulness meditation group two times during the spring and fall every year, and 8–10 Cambodian adult clients have been participating in the group. The group has been run the same way as it was designed with 12 sessions, and the facilitators monitor how the participants understand and utilize meditation in daily life and modify the schedule and level of meditation practice as appropriate for the participants.

Since the beginning of the program, just over 100 patients have participated in the full meditation program.

More than 100 families have participated in the clinic/temple-linked wellness program.

Partnership Toward A Khmer Wellness Center

The partnership between the temple and the clinic has helped the temple to develop into a Khmer community "wellness center." Initially the focus of the clinical program was trauma related to the outcomes from the Pol Pot genocide. And the temple's focus was religion. But, in time, the partnership between the clinic and the temple created a synergy that led to focus on other essential issues in the Khmer community.

Through expanding partnership with the temple, the Cambodian program has developed into a multigenerational wellness center. With the temple as host, the mental health clinicians now run family enrichment programs, first 5 (early childhood intervention) programs, and parenting programs. The clinic works with Khmer community members from prenatal through older adult age ranges. Reaching Khmer youth is of paramount importance.

We use the synergistic power of a western-oriented mental health clinic combined with a community-organizing Buddhist temple for maximal outcome in regard to making services relevant and accessible.

The Story of Tith Chan, Social Worker

I was born in a Thailand refugee camp. I have three sisters, one brother, and three half-sisters. My family immigrated to the United States as refugees in 1982. I was 2 years old then. I have lived in San Jose, California, for practically all of my life.

My life in America has been full of challenges and difficulties. I would describe the environment I grew up in as a "concrete jungle," as the neighborhood I grew up in was quite dangerous.

My family and I were extremely impoverished. My mother was an alcoholic. By the time I was age 5, my mother and father separated. Both my mother and father would eventually find new partners. My living arrangement was unstable. I was the youngest and both of my parents wanted custody of me. I would live with my father, siblings, and his partner for one week, and I would live with my mother, her daughter, and her partner for another week. Both of my parents' partners had some mental health difficulties. My mother's partner was an alcoholic and my father's partner may have had a mood disorder. While I was living with my mother and her partner, I was physically abused. I was forced to change my sister's diaper, and when I was not able to do the task, he would physically abuse me and lock me in the closet. My father's partner was always yelling, screaming, and breaking household items. My father found out that I was being abused by my mother's partner, and he permanently took custody of me. Although I was no longer being physically abused, I then had to endure years of psychological abuse from my father's partner. My eldest sister was adopted by a Christian Caucasian family and was not exposed to the stressors that my brother and two older sisters experienced. My second eldest sister had an arranged marriage and never completed ninth grade. My third eldest sister moved out once she turned 18 years old. My brother eventually started to hang around the neighborhood kids and eventually join a gang. I rarely saw my brother at home because he always came home late at night. I suspect that he did not like to be home as I hated being home. School was my sanctuary, as I could escape home for several hours. As I got older, I stayed out longer, as I did not want to come home. I started to get into trouble both at school and in the community at an early age. My brother was my role model. I had low self-esteem. I had lost faith because I prayed to God as a child hundreds of times to make my family problems go away. No matter how much I prayed, things did not change.

By the time I was age 10, my father sent me and my brother to live with my mother's sister and her family because he did not want us to live with him due to his partner, who was emotionally abusive towards my brother and me. My father lived with his partner and another Cambodian family. I would live with my relatives for about 2 years. Then my brother and I moved to a family friend's, where my father rented a room for us. I barely saw my father. The only time I knew of my father's presence was when I came home from school and I saw food sitting on our beds with a note written in broken English "Foods for Tith Theavy eat."

By the age of 11, I started to experiment with alcohol, tobacco, and marijuana. I had no guidance, no structure, and freedom to do as I wish. I had my first tattoo and owned my first gun at age 12. One of my tattoos symbolized the meaning "My Crazy Life" in gang culture. By age 13 I was already abusing marijuana and alcohol. I was also engaging in gang and criminal activity. I was out of control and I did not care if I lived or died. My brother was incarcerated at the state penitentiary for being at a crime scene of a murder. Again, he was my role model.

At age 15 I moved in with my father and his partner. My father's partner had made some changes and living with her was bearable. However, I was in too deep with the gang lifestyle and was not able to leave the gang behind. I delved into drugs further and eventually started to use methamphetamine and crack cocaine. I became addicted to crack cocaine and spent close to 2 years of my life using the drug. Several of my friends were put behind bars for life and several of them died as result of gang activity. I got arrested one month away from my 18th birthday, which might have been a blessing in disguise. I was put on probation and had many court orders to comply with. I attended drug counseling and attended narcotics anonymous. I was the youngest person in the meeting and the stories I heard from the group participants made me think about my life and the direction I was heading towards. I became clean and sober. I went back to school and tried my best. I stopped socializing with my gang friends. I thought about my life and realized that life is sometimes unfair. I also realized that my father and mother did not plan on coming to this country but were forced due to the killing fields. My father and mother did not plan to separate from one another. My family came with nothing but emotional scars from the war. They lost everything they had in Cambodia and now they are in an alien country and are marginalized. I thought to myself if I feel alienated in this country even though I grew up in America and can read and write, imagine what my father and mother are feeling, as they did not grow up here and are not literate. I stopped blaming them for my life problems. I told myself my mother and father did the best with what they had at the moment. My father raised me and he has done his job and now it is my time to do my job. I forgave my parents for what I endured in the past. I was able to beat the odds.

I went on to junior college and transferred to San Jose State University and received a bachelor's degree and eventually a master's degree in social work.

I came to this field of work because of my past life experiences. My parents' unaddressed mental health and social issues have impacted their ability to provide me with the proper upbringing. I know that other Cambodian youths are experiencing similar unfortunate circumstances that I have. My role is to bring hope to the Cambodian youth and help them understand their lives, help empower them, bring guidance, understand who they are as a person and believe in themselves. Furthermore, I help the Cambodian youth understand that sometimes people are dealt a bad hand in life. However, you can still win depending how you play your cards.

The Lotus Thrives

When the monks planted the lotus all those years ago, they did not know whether it would rot or sprout, whether it would dwindle or bloom.

They forged partnerships to ensure the wellness of a traumatized cohort of refugees with unspeakable stories. They have used age-old wisdom to approach modern tragedy. Through cooperation and mutual understanding the temple and the clinic have grown and become more effective.

Almost 10 years after its inception, the clinical operations, wellness programs, and community activities of the clinic and temple are so seamless that it is difficult to remember a time when these groups were exclusive and their functions separate.

The model described in this narrative may seem exclusive and specific to the Khmer experience. But there are general themes that pertain to effective cross-cultural psychiatry work. In order to be clinically effective with a different cultural group, clinicians must have the right connections in the community, effective brokers of the culture, and an understanding of their population's experience. These things cannot come from a textbook or from a classroom. They can only come from dedicated partnership.

Under the California sun in the backyard of the world's technology industry, the Cambodian lotus now blooms in the garden of our temple at Wat Khemara Rangsey.

References

1. Van Schaack B, Reicherter D, Chhang Y, Talbott A. Cambodia's hidden scars: trauma psychology in the wake of the Khmer Rouge. Phnom Penh: Documentation Center of Cambodia Press; 2011.
2. Mollica RF, Wyshak G, Lavelle J. The psychosocial impact of war trauma and torture on southeast Asian refugees. Am J Psychiatry. 1987;144:1567–72.
3. Saechao F, Sharrock S, Reicherter D, Livingston JD, Aylward A, Whisnant J, et al. Stressors and barriers to utilizing mental health services among diverse groups of first-generation immigrants to the United States. Community Ment Health J. 2012;48:98–106.
4. Reicherter D, Venerable Rong Be. Mindfulness meditation after trauma. In: Khmer Krom Journey to Self Determination. Khmer Krom Federation, December 2009.
5. American Psychiatric Association. Diagnostic and statistical manual of mental disorders. 4th ed. Washington, DC: American Psychiatry Publishing; 1994.
6. Silove D, Manicavasagar V, Mollica R, Thai M, Khiek D, Lavelle J, et al. Screening for depression and PTSD in a Cambodian population unaffected by war: comparing the Hopkins Symptom Checklist and Harvard Trauma Questionnaire with the structured clinical interview. J Nerv Ment Dis. 2007;195:152–7.
7. Hinton DE, Hinton AL, Eng KT, Choung S. PTSD and key somatic complaints and cultural syndromes among rural Cambodians: the results of a needs assessment survey. Med Anthropol Q. 2012;26:383–407.
8. Han M, Valencia M, Lee Y, De Leon J. Development and implementation of the culturally competent program with Cambodians: the pilot psycho-social-cultural treatment group program. J Ethn Cultur Divers Soc Work. 2012;21:212–30.

Narrative 5
Kombis, Brothels, and Violence Against Women: Building Global Health Partnerships to Address Women's Health and Empowerment

Christina Tara Khan

This is a story of an early-career physician-scholar's experiences in academic-community partnerships in Peru, in work focused on cultivating a public health approach to girls' and women's empowerment in communities.

My year as a Fogarty research fellow was a formative experience on my path to promoting girls' and women's health. I was 27 years old and somewhat green as far as public health fieldwork internationally. I had spent time in Latin America studying medicine and community health but usually in formal health settings, such as health centers or hospitals. I was passionate about empowering vulnerable populations and had spent several years working in health education and promotion with special population groups at the university during my doctoral studies in community health. I had not yet worked with a population as marginalized as sex workers, nor had I done research in the area of violence against women. Per the suggestion of a good friend, I applied for the National Institutes of Health-Fogarty Ellison International Clinical Research Scholars Fellowship, an auspicious career move that would take me to Peru to learn about and conduct studies in global health and clinical research.

C.T. Khan, M.D., Ph.D. (✉)
Department of Psychiatry and Behavioral Sciences, Stanford University School
of Medicine and Veterans Affairs Palo Alto Health Care System, Stanford, CA, USA
e-mail: ckhan@stanford.edu

© Springer International Publishing Switzerland 2015
L.W. Roberts et al. (eds.), *Partnerships for Mental Health*,
DOI 10.1007/978-3-319-18884-3_5

Fogarty Fellowship in Peru

During my fellowship year, I designed two primary research projects: one epidemiological study looking at cervical cancer survival rates at the Peruvian National Cancer Institute and the other an offshoot of a community-based prevention project for human immunodeficiency virus and sexually transmitted infections. The prevention project was taking place in communities around Peru, targeting both the general population and specific vulnerable groups, including female and male commercial sex workers. Early in my fellowship year I had the opportunity to travel and participate in the project in the Andean and Amazonian regions of Peru, where the resources were scarcer than in Lima but the communities smaller and tighter. I had grown up and lived mostly in small cities or metropolitan areas, and these trips opened my eyes to the realities of poverty in more isolated parts of the world. In many ways these regions were reminiscent of my parents' native Guyana, which is also largely impoverished and shares borders on the Amazon. I was eager to see and learn as much as I could during that year.

Despite 4 months of gastrointestinal upset that accompanied my initial stay in Peru and earned me the nickname "Typhoid Christina," I was in a global-health-minded-medical-student's paradise. Public health fieldwork and research in South America is what I had aspired to do since my undergraduate years, and I was finally there for a solid stretch of time. Back in Lima, I began working in a clinic that served sex workers at a community health center in Callao, a port city adjoining the sprawling metropolis of Lima. Callao for me was a city of contrasts, being both an epicenter for Afro-Peruvian salsa dancing and a neighborhood that had seen better days, now characterized by row after row of abandoned warehouses. Often taxi drivers would not want to take me to the health center, claiming the neighborhood was too *peligroso* (dangerous). If I couldn't find a cab, I would take the Kombi, an old, often dilapidated Volkswagen van painted a unique style and combination of colors to designate the route, and blasting salsa or reggaeton music along the way. Whereas the taxi would cost about 5 US dollars, the Kombi charged about 15 cents to go from the closest Lima neighborhood to the neighborhood where the health center was located. My expat colleagues warned me not to take the bus and walk through the neighborhood alone, due to the frequent crime that occurred in close proximity to the health center. Being a *morena* (brown) gringa, I took my chances and fortunately was safe during these trips (I later ended up getting mugged when I was alone in a taxi in another part of Lima).

Community Health

At the health center, I did a combination of clinical observation and health promotion work. Early on, I mostly observed and shadowed various staff: the clinic's director (a physician), the social worker, and the head *promotoras* (peer educators).

We worked both in the clinic at the health center and in a mobile clinic van, in which we frequented bars, nightclubs, and brothels in outreach to the clientele. In the smaller cities of the Amazon region, we also visited barbershops, salons, and hotels, which were common meeting points for the workers and their clientele. It was true community health, wherein we as health workers went out into the field to offer primary and secondary prevention based on evidence-based health science. In this particular case, we were offering testing for sexually transmitted infections, counseling, and, if necessary, treatment, in exchange for the sex workers' time and their trust. It was a relationship that demanded a certain level of trust due to the disruptions it caused to their work. We tried to be discreet, but there was little way to hide that our group of health workers was not part of the regular scene.

Conditions in the bars, hotels, and brothels were substandard: often a grimy back room with a bed, very poor lighting, and nowhere to wash hands. With the street workers, the exchange was sometimes done in a motel they used for work. We always offered condoms and sometimes lubricant, for which they were ever grateful. Often the exchange was quick but always there was a sharing of greetings and well wishing. The mobile team was well known and liked by their clientele. During the visits, the clinic director would patiently explain to me what she was doing and her strategy for outreach. We talked about how it could be hard to do follow-up given the transient nature of the population, with frequent moves from site to site either to find work or for safety. I heard story after story about how these women were maltreated—by their clients, by the owners of the establishments in which they worked, by their own partners and families, and even by the police. Oh, so often by the police, and by other law enforcement officials. I heard sad and appalling stories about women being beaten, assaulted, and on the run, constantly hypervigilant to the dangers that lurked around them. They occupied a space between high demand—in a society where utilization of commercial sex work was frequent—and lowest regard—in a primarily Catholic country where they were shamed for their "dirty" profession. A country where rates of violence against women were among the highest in the world [1] and, although there were no known statistics at the time, where I suspected sex workers were even more vulnerable to gender-based violence. There were many contradictions that I tried hard to understand but could not.

The brothels in Callao were larger than I ever could have imagined. Picture an abandoned warehouse with room after room dedicated to commercial sex work. The cars would start lining up in the early evening, and men would filter in an out, as if it were a factory. The place was heavily guarded at the front, although there was much less security in the areas where the women were working. The rooms were dimly lit with a bed and a sink and very little else. Each woman had a few things in the room, including some tissues, her stash of protection, occasionally a flower or decoration to give the room some color. I remember feeling curious, surprised, and saddened to see the conditions the women worked in. I was disillusioned to find out that some of the women were as young as 18 years old, perhaps even younger. It seemed not right, but I tried not to let my own judgments and beliefs get in the way of the work we were there to do. We were there to provide a service, to help maintain these women's sexual and reproductive health, despite the conditions they were working in. I heard stories of clients not wanting to use protection and using various tactics to achieve this goal. Some offered more money; others used violence or coercion. Some of the sex workers were okay with taking more money; others refused to practice without protection. Rules were few and violations were common.

Over the next 3 years, I established a relationship with this population that eventually led to the privilege of learning more in-depth about their experiences. The relationship building began with the clinic and mobile visits and was enhanced by several community events at the health center, to commemorate the anniversary of a program or to celebrate a national holiday. I regularly attended these events if I was able, enjoying the opportunity to get to know the clients and the health center staff "off hours." Often there was music and dancing, and as a salsa aficionado, I came to be known as "Doctora Salsera." The sharing of music and dance went beyond just appreciation of the arts. I believe it helped to create a common bond that revealed the human behind the roles we each held. It helped us to feel connected on a level that is important for establishing safety. I believe it played a crucial role in the development of rapport and trust, and it helped me to feel even more acutely the unjust and painful experiences these women had undergone and continued to face in their daily lives. I was inspired to better understand gender-based violence and to try to promote empowerment around human rights.

Researching Violence Against Female Sex Workers

In collaboration with the health center workers and the *promotoras*, I developed a screening tool to assess the sex workers' experience of violence. We ran a pilot focus group where we explored the types of violence these women faced and discussed what constitutes violence against women. Astonishingly, I learned that many women had assumed certain types of violence as integral to their role as wives. Later on I would learn that this was a common phenomenon in many parts of the world, not just in Peru. We talked about human rights and their rights as women and as sex workers. These discussions were moving both for me and for the participants, many of whom learned they were not alone in their struggle. The women expressed appreciation for the opportunity to have a voice, and I, too, was empowered in my efforts to give voice to what I was learning was an overwhelming suffering in silence.

I decided to design a formal research study, to expose these injustices and share what I was learning with others. At this point my fellowship year was nearing its end, and I knew the approval would not come through before I returned to the United States. The study required approval from various entities, including the health center board and *promotora* group and the institutional review boards where my mentors worked, at the Universidad Nacional Mayor de San Marcos and the University of Washington. Extensive paperwork and many reminder e-mails finally got things through, an approval process that was more detailed than usual due to the international setting, cross-institutional research, and an especially vulnerable population.

In the 2 years that intervened, I returned to Peru approximately once per year during my time off, to maintain contact with my colleagues, the health center staff, and my Peruvian "family" and friends. Two years after the planning process for the research study had begun, I came upon a fortuitous break in residency training and the opportunity to conduct the focus group study.

For the formal study, we held four focus groups: two each with small groups of street-based and brothel-based sex workers, to capture the disparate experiences each group faced in their home and work environments. The head *promotoras* at the clinic helped with recruitment, and I trained them to facilitate the focus groups. We conducted the groups in different places, according to convenience and safety for the group participants, some at the Universidad Nacional Mayor de San Marcos, others in the homes of the *promotoras*. This time around I was a few years removed from my regular presence in the clinic; I knew the promotoras who had been working for years with the clinic but did not recognize many of the group participants.

Initially in each group there was some hesitation and silence. Feeling self-conscious, I wondered if, in part, this had to do with me being a foreigner who spoke Spanish with an accent. In retrospect, more likely it had to do with our asking them to disclose private and intimate details about their lives and their work with regard to a topic that was rarely discussed, gender-based violence. In each group we began with introductions and telling a little about ourselves. The women shared how long they had been working in their respective locales, and I shared my background and experiences working at the health center and on the mobile team. We provided a meal and drinks to help create a comfortable atmosphere. It was not long into the discussions that it seemed the ice had broken and participants began to speak more freely. It began to feel as if I had known the women from my previous time at the clinic. The familiarity of the *promotoras* and the clinic social worker helped; these were women they knew and trusted with their health concerns. By the end of the groups, all manner of hesitation seemed to have dissolved, the women were speaking openly, and many of the participants wanted to take pictures together. In a heartwarming gesture, one of the participants took off her earrings and offered them to me as a gift, stating she wanted to share with me something to remember her and the others when I return to the United States. Her kindness towards someone who before that day had been a complete stranger was tremendous.

Lessons Learned

This was the first community-based study I had implemented in an international setting. The process unfolded over several years, and though this may not be ideal for the publishing demands of academia, it was conducive to the development of a partnership involving trust. In each community I have worked in before and since, trust has been the most important ingredient for fostering a strong relationship. It is the foundation of an academic-community partnership, without which our "data" may be invalid, or biased, at best.

I was fortunate to have had, through this trust, the opportunity to learn about a different reality, one that a large proportion of the world's women face and from which no woman is immune, regardless of nationality, profession, income, or race. While the findings of the study are shared elsewhere, the lessons I learned through this process keenly shaped my path as a researcher and clinician. The women involved in the study also expressed gratitude for the opportunity to partake. They were appreciative of a forum to express their concerns and share their experiences with their peers. They learned about their rights as women and gained insight into the daily injustices they and their colleagues faced, not only by virtue of their profession but sometimes merely because of their gender. Armed with this knowledge, the women bravely participate in organizations focused on justice, including sex worker unions and activist groups. They bring their concerns to events such as the women's march on the *Día Internacional de la Mujer* (International Day of the Woman), in which I was privileged to participate. These events bring airtime about these issues to local media outlets and contribute to the slow process of cultural shift, a process that begins with awareness and education.

The beauty of academic-community partnerships lies in this potential for a mutually sought-out process. Researchers who seek to advance knowledge and improve social conditions may share with a community who is also seeking improvement in social conditions the theoretical and practical lessons learned from research. Through careful and thoughtful collaboration, the research team and the community begin the process of building trust. From there develops the potential for designing or adapting interventions to target deep-rooted social inequities such as gender-based violence. Although the evidence base on prevention of violence against women is young, particularly in low- and middle-income countries, there are many promising strategies, all of which begin with a community alliance [2]. To address multifaceted problems such as gender-based violence, a public health approach is needed, and communities around the world are implementing strategies in collaboration with academic and multi-sector agencies.

Because of my experiences in Peru, as well as other times spent among women and girls in Zimbabwe and Zambia, my work is now focused on cultivating a public health approach to girls and women's empowerment in communities around the globe. I believe it is through the commonalities we share rather than our differences that we are able to foster trust in academic-community partnerships and promote the acquisition of knowledge and skills needed to bring about change. As Nobel Laureate Leymah Gbowee remarked regarding hope and the potential for change, "Will you journey with me to help that girl, be it an African girl, or an American girl, or a Japanese girl... to fulfill her wish, fulfill her dream, achieve that dream... Let's journey together, let's journey together" [3].

> "*I believe it is through the commonalities we share rather than our differences that we are able to foster trust in academic-community partnerships and promote the acquisition of knowledge and skills needed to bring about change.*"

References

1. World Health Organization. WHO multi-country study on women's health and domestic violence against women: initial results on prevalence, health outcomes, and women's responses. Geneva: World Health Organization; 2005.
2. World Health Organization/London School of Hygiene and Tropical Medicine. Preventing intimate partner and sexual violence against women: taking action and generating evidence. Geneva: World Health Organization; 2010.
3. Gbowee L. Unlock the intelligence, passion, greatness of girls. March, 2012. Available at http://www.ted.com/talks/leymah_gbowee_unlock_the_intelligence_passion_greatness_of_girls?language=en.

Narrative 6
Creating a National Native Telebehavioral Health Network: The IHS Telebehavioral Health Center of Excellence

Steven Adelsheim, Caroline Bonham, Chris Fore, Joe Glass, Dorlynn Simmons, and Leonard Thomas

This is a story of several health care leaders with the objective of providing care for tribal communities, who forged academic-community partnerships to establish a National Native Telebehavioral Health Network.

The views and opinions expressed in this narrative are those of the authors and do not necessarily represent the official position of the Indian Health Service.

S. Adelsheim, M.D. (✉)
Department of Psychiatry and Behavioral Sciences, Stanford University School of Medicine, Stanford, CA, USA
e-mail: sadelsheim@stanford.edu

C. Bonham, M.D., M.S.
Department of Psychiatry and Behavioral Sciences, University of New Mexico Health Sciences Center, Albuquerque, NM, USA
e-mail: cbonham@salud.unm.edu

C. Fore, Ph.D.
Department of Behavioral Health, Indian Health Service Telebehavioral Health Center of Excellence, Albuquerque, NM, USA
e-mail: chris.fore@ihs.gov

J. Glass, M.S.
Department of Behavioral Health, Mescalero Indian Hospital, Mescalero, NM, USA

D. Simmons, M.S.S.W.
Mescalero Service Unit, Mescalero, NM, USA
e-mail: dorlynn.simmons@ihs.gov

L. Thomas, M.D.
Indian Health Service, Albuquerque Area Office, Albuquerque, NM, USA
e-mail: leonard.thomas@ihs.gov

© Springer International Publishing Switzerland 2015
L.W. Roberts et al. (eds.), *Partnerships for Mental Health*,
DOI 10.1007/978-3-319-18884-3_6

Pam's New Shoes

Pam was a 12-year-old girl living in a rural, tribal community who had been retained one year in school and likely had been socially promoted to the seventh grade. Her school record was minimal but reflected deficiencies in both academics and social adjustment. She wore glasses with thick lenses, which seemed to magnify the size of her eyes, and she appeared to have recently gone through her adolescent growth spurt, which left her thin and wiry with long gangly limbs. It also left her with behavior that was at times aggressive and undercontrolled. In fact, she was referred to Joe Glass of the local Behavioral Health Service after being suspended for physically hitting a teacher. The school felt that Pam's behavior was a complete enigma, and most of the faculty was wary of her and concerned for their safety. Mr. Glass did an initial interview and screening that suggested multiple problems, including low academic achievement and behavioral issues. Pam's speech was markedly slow but seemed very deliberate, and she had a very dry and rather subtle sense of humor that seemed a little odd. Mr. Glass had been working with a child psychiatrist, Dr. Steve Adelsheim, in an early telehealth partnership with the University of New Mexico, and together they decided to try to get as many of the people and agencies possible together to get a better understanding and possibly develop a plan to help Pam.

The school stated that Pam's grandmother, who was raising Pam and several other grandchildren, had not been to the school building, but they could send out a community family liaison worker to explain the plan, invite her to the meeting if she approved and get the permissions and releases signed. Her grandmother did approve and signed the documents. On the day of the meeting she did not come, but several of Pam's teachers, her counselor, the middle school principal, the school nurse, the school contract psychologist, and a representative of a family support agency who had visited the family in the home met with Mr. Glass and Dr. Adelsheim via telehealth. A much clearer picture of Pam's academic achievement and her often erratic and inconsistent behavior, along with a better understanding of her social and family situation, developed. Pam would often just walk out of classes and never participated in any physical education activities. A complete educational assessment was scheduled within weeks instead of months. During the session it seemed that the instructional staff felt rather alienated from Pam, but she had a more positive, or at least neutral, contact with the school nurse. One of the things the nurse had noticed was that Pam's tennis shoes were worn out with tears and holes and broken shoelaces; she could barely walk in them. The principal knew of a service club that would give students in need a voucher of up to $30 for shoes, and the family advocacy agency arranged to get the voucher and take Pam to buy a pair of new shoes.

Pam began seeing the school counselor and continued sessions with Mr. Glass and Dr. Adelsheim. She agreed if she had to leave the classroom the school nurse would be notified and she would go to the health clinic, where she could sit and the nurse would interact with her as time allowed. The educational evaluation did further define learning disabilities, and she was eligible for special education services. While resources and even her participation were improving, Pam continued to be isolated from the instructional staff and other students. Her physical education coach agreed that if Pam did not want to participate in class activities, she could walk or run around the football field, and run she did. The coach said that she was amazed that Pam would run the entire period, and indeed she was a fast runner, a really fast runner. Pam's school athletic department was having what is euphemistically called building years, but in fact it meant they had very little to brag about in the sports program. Pam had caught the attention of the coaching staff. They encouraged Pam and then accompanied her to the regional Special Olympics, where she won first place in distance events as well as placed in other running events. She was invited to the state Special Olympics and, though not winning first place, came home with several awards. The result of this was that Pam bonded with teachers and some students and probably for the first time, just for a pair of running shoes, had a sense of belonging and enjoyment at school. Pam will have challenges for the rest of her life, but she now had the experience and ability to meet those challenges in a totally different manner. The telehealth program demonstrated the power of being able to quickly bring together a number of caring adults from the environment of a 12-year-old girl and the effectiveness of even a single meeting to make an important difference in her life.

Defining the Issue

Providing high quality and effective mental health and substance abuse services to a geographically isolated population is an ongoing challenge throughout the United States. With the increasing number of people eligible for mental health and substance abuse services (which, for the purposes of this narrative, we will combine to call "behavioral health" services) due to the Affordable Care Act and parity, the ongoing lack of a strong workforce to meet the demand for service only increases the number of people with difficulty accessing behavioral health services. In addition, the stigma and blame surrounding acknowledgement that one faces mental health challenges makes ongoing advocacy for expanded services more difficult. In rural and frontier communities these many factors lead to overwhelming difficulty in ensuring access to critical mental health care. Within New Mexico, where over half the state's counties are designated as rural or frontier (less than 6 people per square mile), many of these isolated counties and communities are the ancestral homes to some of the 22 tribes that make up New Mexico's Native American communities. In other cases, these remote communities are reservation lands that tribes have come to live on more recently as a result of complex interactions with the federal government.

The Indian Health Service (IHS), an agency within the Department of Health and Human Services, is responsible for providing federal health services to Native Americans and Alaska Natives. The IHS is the principal federal health care provider and health advocate for Native American people, and its goal is to raise health status to the highest possible level. IHS provides a comprehensive health service delivery system for approximately 1.9 million Native Americans who belong to 564 federally recognized tribes in 35 states. IHS is staffed predominantly by Native Americans, and regional area offices or local service units are often closely tied to the community they serve. Employees have a personal understanding of the needs of the community, and familiarity with culturally appropriate treatment, prevention, and education. Significant health disparities exist for urban Native American populations [1], including tremendous underfunding of services in tribal communities [2]. Whereas more than 50 % of Native Americans do not use substances, many American Indians and Alaska Natives continue to struggle with substance use disorders [3]. The suicide rate among American Indians and Alaska Native under age 25 for all US counties is approximately 3.5 times the national average for Whites of the same age [4]. Yet, despite these risk factors, considerable strengths also exist in Native American communities. Many Native Americans have an especially strong sense of community connectedness, cultural identity, and family and social support, which are all protective factors for wellness [5].

Introducing the Partners

The IHS Tele-behavioral Health Center of Excellence (TBHCE) was created through a partnership between the Albuquerque Area of the Indian Health Service (AAIHS) and the University of New Mexico (UNM) Department of Psychiatry and Behavioral Sciences Center for Rural and Community Behavioral Health (CRCBH). The AAIHS is one of 12 area offices of the IHS. The AAIHS is responsible for the provision of health services in New Mexico to 19 Pueblos; the Jicarilla and Mescalero Apaches; and the Alamo, To'hajiilee, and Ramah Chapters of the Navajo Nation. In addition, the AAIHS also serves the Southern Ute and the Ute Mountain Ute Reservations in southern Colorado; the Ysleta Del Sur Pueblo in El Paso, Texas; and two Urban Indian Centers, located in Albuquerque, New Mexico, and Denver, Colorado. The CRCBH was developed through the Department of Psychiatry and Behavioral Sciences at the UNM School of Medicine, with a mission to address "health care disparities through: education and workforce development; health services research and evaluation; capacity building; and through increasing access to quality behavioral health services that are holistic, cost-effective and provided with respect to the unique cultures within the communities of New Mexico" [6].

The birth of the TBHCE came from discussions between Leonard Thomas, M.D., chief medical officer (CMO) for the AAIHS, and Steven Adelsheim, M.D., director of the CRCBH. In his role as CMO, Dr. Thomas, in partnership with the tribes within the AAIHS, had been facing the complex issues that emerged from the lack of mental health supports and services across the region with many tribes. Dr. Thomas and Dr. Adelsheim began to discuss the need for expanded access to child mental health support for the tribal partners within the AAIHS. Both had become interested in the promise of telehealth through discussions taking place with the creation of the New Mexico Telehealth Commission, of which Dr. Adelsheim had become a commissioner, and through a workgroup of Dr. Thomas, focused on developing a grant to the Federal Communications Commission to expand communication and telehealth connectivity throughout rural communities in New Mexico.

Getting Started

During the 2006 New Mexico legislative session, the state Telehealth Commission promoted funding to create a pilot program at the UNM School of Medicine focusing on early intervention support for children and adolescents across the areas of developmental disabilities, obesity prevention, and suicide prevention. The suicide prevention pilot funds of $40,000 were distributed to the CRCBH, and Dr. Adelsheim approached Dr. Thomas to consider using these funds to initiate a child/ adolescent tele-behavioral health pilot with interested AAIHS partners. The initial response from the behavioral health directors of the eight regional "service units" was negative, because major concerns were raised about the technological limitations of telehealth. In addition, service unit directors noted the potential expansion of an already-existing cultural divide that might come from being seen for mental health services by a non-Native provider, with the additional barriers of technology and distance. Furthermore, there was some skepticism about partnering with the local university, which had a reputation with many tribal partners of having faculty who came to communities with a promise of support and services, only to be present on a short-term basis to obtain information for research or to start a short-term program to support academic promotion and then leave. Initially no site expressed interest in participating in the pilot. Ultimately after several meetings where the potential pilot was repeatedly raised by Dr. Thomas, the Mescalero Apache Service Unit agreed to give the model a try.

The Mescalero Apache Service Unit is in a remote part of southern New Mexico, requiring a 3.5-hour drive to Albuquerque, New Mexico, to access most specialty care. The facility had been without psychiatric services for several years, after the death of their long-time psychiatric care provider. The hospital had five primary care providers addressing patients' medical and behavioral health needs. The providers at Mescalero wanted psychiatric support and consultation to help them manage complex co-occurring disorders and serious mental illness. In addition, the Service Unit had never had child psychiatric services as a treatment option. Joe Glass, M.S., was the behavioral health program director who had been working in community mental health centers since the beginning of the movement in the 1960s and had committed his whole career to building a range of community-based supports for those from health disparity populations. Mr. Glass began to see the potential of the telehealth program as a way to link needed services to the Mescalero community while also providing him with a collaborative partnership that could help prevent burnout and the isolation he felt as the sole provider. Together with Dorlynn Simmons, the chief executive officer at the Mescalero Apache Service Unit, a Mescalero tribal leader, and a long-time social worker, a plan came about to support the initiative.

Towards an Approach/Solution

Although Mr. Glass knew there was a strong need for this initiative, he was initially quite uncertain as to the potential for its success. Mr. Glass did not think he would work well with an "academician" because work in rural and remote communities is so different from academic medical centers. He was concerned Dr. Adelsheim would not have the flexibility and creativity required to provide care in such a rural, impoverished community. In addition, when Mr. Glass heard about the need for the contracts for communication across agencies, credentialing agreements for the providers, consent forms for telehealth, and the protocols required for developing the service, he guessed that legal barriers might prevent the program from ever getting off the ground. The agreements did percolate through the systems, however, and using telehealth equipment that had been distributed to service units, Mr. Glass and Dr. Adelsheim decided to test out the model with one client whom they decided to see together, with Mr. Glass in the Mescalero Hospital conference room and Dr. Adelsheim in the AAIHS conference room 216 miles away.

The initial visit seemed to go well, and Mr. Glass found that even though Dr. Adelsheim was an "academic," he had a disarming way of approaching people that left people feeling comfortable, and he decided they could work together. Over time, administrative processes for scheduling and recordkeeping came together, allowing for the team to begin increasing services. Eventually services were provided a half day per week. It was a great partnership. Because of his long-term relationships with many generations of family members within the Mescalero community, Mr. Glass could provide critical clinical and historical context before

Joe knew that ultimately the tele-video partnership would work for Mescalero. He had previously worked at one of the first community mental health centers in Texas, which had a team consultation model of multiple consultants meeting with a patient together to figure out what was needed to support that individual. Joe's sense was that clients always appreciated the focus of more providers trying to be of support and, rather than feeling intimidated by all the people in the room, they appreciated everyone's effort to be helpful together. Joe then had gone to work at Mescalero and been there 17 years, working with many generations of family members from across the community. Joe sensed that the telehealth model would be seen in a similar way to the team consultations in Texas. He framed the visit video sessions by telling people they were going to be on TV with a doctor from the university who was an expert and would help figure out how to help the person feel better. He told folks that even though the doc was hundreds of miles away, after a few minutes it would feel like the doc was right there with them. Joe encouraged people to just try it for a few minutes and that he would be right there with them to be of support and they could stop the visit if they didn't like it. Afterwards people would tell Joe the whole thing was amazing and that it was just like the doc was right there in the room with them.

each visit and clear questions to be addressed in the shared interview. Dr. Adelsheim could provide clinical guidance in terms of assessment, therapeutic direction, and medical support for Mr. Glass' interventions. When medications were needed, Mr. Glass would pass the prescription information from Dr. Adelsheim to one of the Mescalero primary care providers, who wrote the script for the patient. Eventually, the IHS team made a larger commitment to this effort and created a new video studio and linked the new electronic health record (EHR) Mr. Glass was working on to the telehealth network. The EHR allowed the psychiatrists in Albuquerque to see the notes from the Mescalero providers, then put their notes directly into the medical record of the patient, and write prescriptions directly into the IHS system. Soon an addictionologist joined the team, and services were able to expand.

Expanding the Partnership

Mr. Glass and Dr. Adelsheim continued telehealth services at Mescalero. It became clear to Mr. Glass that this model was very important when he saw the surprised reaction of other service unit leaders when he went to meetings and told them how Mescalero now had 4 hours per week of child psychiatry service and 4 hours per week of pain/addictions services. Eventually other services units joined up, as well as other UNM psychiatrists. The benefits in terms of expanded access to clinical service were seen as valuable, and UNM had the additional benefit of expanded partnership in a whole new venue with a critical community partner. Eventually schools were connected to various sites through a telehealth bridge through IHS in South Dakota, allowing for three-way connections with clinic, school, and UNM. These school connections became an additional, regularly scheduled part of the telepsychiatry system. They proved especially valuable when the state of New Mexico put out a call to tribal communities to participate in a federal youth suicide prevention grant application. When Mr. Glass heard about the announcement from Dr. Adelsheim, he immediately contacted his CEO, Ms. Simmons, and the Mescalero School superintendent. Within an hour, all were on a video connection discussing how to work with the state to apply for the grant, which was ultimately successful and served the school and community for 3 years.

Around this time, Dr. Fore, who had previously worked for IHS as a psychologist with the Acoma-Canoncito-Laguna service unit, returned to the AAIHS as the behavioral health consultant. Dr. Adelsheim and Mr. Glass shared with him the work being done via televideo, and Dr. Fore was interested in expanding the telehealth model. Together they began to expand services to other service units in the AAIHS. When the IHS headquarters office released a funding announcement for the development of a telebehavioral health center, the team quickly put together a proposal that laid out the development of the existing model into a regional telebehavioral health hub. With the success of this application, the IHS Telebehavioral Health Center of Excellence (TBHCE) was created.

Growth

Dr. Fore started to build the IHS TBHCE along with Dr. Caroline Bonham, who managed the program from the CRCBH side. They approached local community providers to understand their priorities and needs regarding access to behavioral health care. The AAIHS office collaborated with UNM on a formal needs assessment with local community providers. These conversations most commonly revolved around access to care, leading to the realization that there were two ways the TBHCE and CRCBH could increase access: through clinical care and through distant education.

Clinical Care

By providing direct telebehavioral health services, access to care has increased significantly. What started with Mr. Glass and Dr. Adelsheim at one site now involves 19 sites across the United States (Fig. 6.1).

Services grew from child psychiatry to adult psychiatry, addictions psychiatry, geriatric psychiatry, and infant mental health psychiatry. As with the initial development of services in Mescalero, the establishment of each new clinical site required regular communication with multiple stakeholders to clarify mutual roles, expectations, and responsibilities and to build relationships and trust over e-mail, phone, and video conferencing. On the basis of numerous community requests, the Center provided adult, child,

The three-way connection between the Mescalero clinic, Mescalero School, and UNM Telehealth became a really important way to support students and their families when issues arose at school. As a tribal school, Mescalero School had great leadership and wonderful educators but was underresourced in support for students with major needs. The televideo connection was especially helpful in supporting students with mental health issues who were in special education. In one case, a student was being kept out of class for behavioral issues and working with the janitor as an effort to develop vocational skills; with the televideo collaboration, a new strategy was developed through behavioral health and medication support to help the student stay in class successfully and get back on track. For a student with intellectual disabilities who was overmedicated, everyone could collaborate on ways to help the young man taper down to a safer dose of medication, which would also allow him to be more aware, alert, and involved with his school program. The telehealth program was especially helpful for students with school phobia. They could meet with the school folks via video with mental health support and make a plan to transition back to school with strong support.

and family telecounseling. Overall, during fiscal year 2013, service hours were up 61 % and patient contacts were up 62 % as compared to the previous year. All told, in fiscal year 2013 more than 4500 patients were seen during 2878 hours of service. Despite these successes, the team realized that this solution did not scale up care

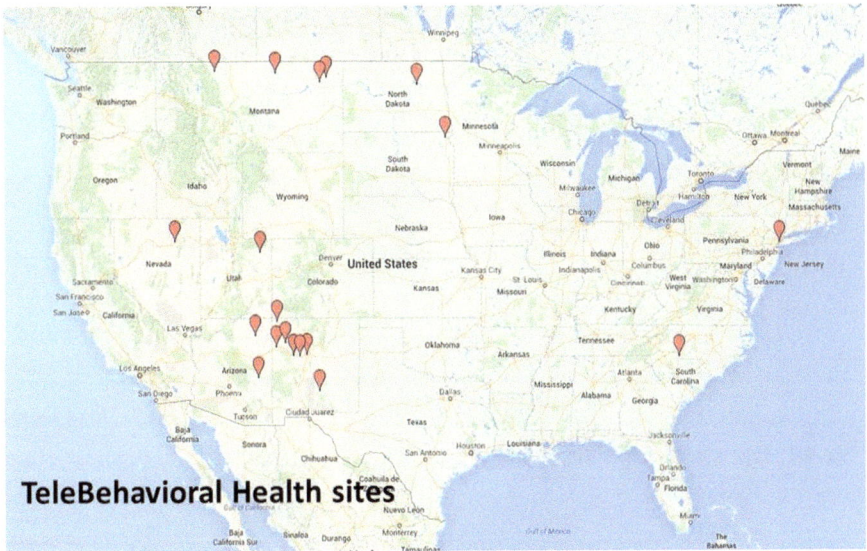

Fig. 6.1 Current clinical sites receiving telehealth services through IHS TBHCE

quickly enough to meet the need. Given the now national scope of the program and the expanded interest in it, additional methods for increasing access were needed.

Distance Education

It became clear that adding a tele-education program for providers working in IHS and tribal rural/frontier clinics would also increase access to care. Through these educational opportunities, rural and frontier providers would have increased capacity and confidence in providing care to those with more complex behavioral health conditions and have a system for additional consultation and training as necessary. After several unsuccessful trials using regular face-to-face video connections, the decision was made to switch to a Web-based learning system. Although this change proved to be challenging, time has shown it to be the correct choice. Growth within this tele-learning community was extraordinary. Hourlong webinars were now provided on behavioral health topics routinely encountered in primary care and behavioral health clinics, as well as sessions on crisis management and risk assessment. Most of the presenters were from CRCBH and represent clinicians and public health professionals from a broad interdisciplinary background with experience working in rural and Native American communities. The focus of the seminars has been to provide specific and pragmatic information with a culturally sensitive approach for providers working in rural/frontier area communities serving Native Americans. Dr. Fore facilitated the majority of these sessions using a conversational and

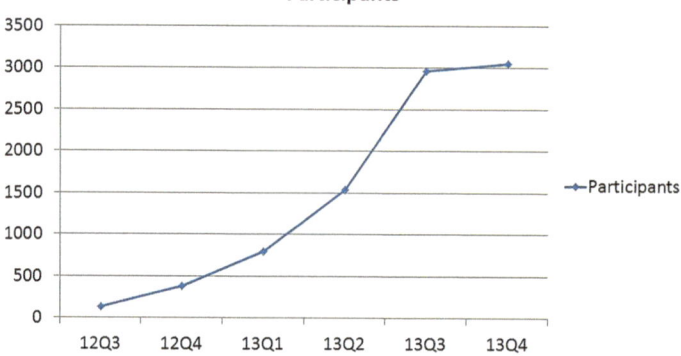

Fig. 6.2 Tele-education totals over time

interactive approach to encourage participation and critical thinking from attendees. Learners were encouraged to use the online chat and survey functions to engage with the presenters during the webinars. In addition to providing current clinical information on behavioral health, the interactive nature of these webinars helped to develop a sense of community among providers working in rural and isolated settings. During the first quarter of the program (fiscal year 2012, quarter 3), 135 providers were trained. During the last quarter of fiscal year 2013, 3050 providers were trained, an increase of 2260 % in 16 months (Fig. 6.2). During fiscal year 2013, the 156 educational seminars held trained more than 8700 providers, and more than 5000 free continuing medical education (CME) credits and continuing education units (CEUs) were provided.

Outcomes

Within the clinical telebehavioral program we have noted that patients are 2.5 times more likely to come for their telepsychiatry appointment than an "in-person" psychiatry session. This is particularly surprising given that they have to travel to the clinic for either type of session. When asked about this, the vast majority of patients said they feel that the telepsychiatry session is more confidential than "in-person." They know that they will not run into their provider at the local school or grocery store and therefore feel that the chances of confidentiality breaches are less. Although the telecounseling component is relatively new, there is also strong anecdotal evidence to support it. For example, during the first 2 weeks of the program the psychologist was told by three different women, "If you were in the room I wouldn't tell you this." All three then went on to disclose histories of childhood sexual abuse, which were extremely relevant to the treatment.

Given that the Native American population is the most impoverished in the US [7], it is important to consider the benefits for our patients. In fiscal year 2013, due to telebehavioral health services, IHS patients avoided 500,000+ miles of travel, which translates into $305,000+ in cost savings for them. Because of the telebehavioral health program, our patients did not miss 16,450+ hours of work/school.

To claim CME/CEUs through the tele-education program, a brief survey must be completed. This has yielded some interesting information. When asked if the Web-based training increased their confidence in their clinical abilities, 93 % agreed. Ninety-five percent reported that they would incorporate the seminar materials into their clinical practice.

Reflections on Lessons Learned

Starting small really does work. It is amazing for all involved to consider how a half day per week child psychiatry pilot between CRCBH and Mescalero turned into a national telebehavioral health center within 5 years. Taking the time to develop an effective model right up front really can speed expansion over time.

Bureaucracy can be conquered and persistence pays off. The processes for developing clinical agreements, funding contracts, and credentialing all took amazing amounts of persistence and dedication on the part of many. A large amount of hope and persistence, combined with dedicated leadership at the top, allowed for these critical components to be completed.

Telehealth takes a champion on each end of the camera. Each telehealth site is only as successful as the champions on each end of the camera. Particularly on the patient site, administrative support and a clinical champion were necessary to clear bureaucracy, find the equipment, create a space, and build the model.

Follow the community's lead. In each successful telebehavioral health site, the type of start-up services, the model, and systems were determined by community need. Had the academic center driven the process, the model would just not have expanded.

Community-academic partnerships should be joined with an eye to the long term. One example of this is the long-term partnership that ultimately developed between the Mescalero Service Unit and CRCBH. Since the telehealth partnership began, the programs have worked together to receive and implement a SAMHSA Systems of Care grant, a SAMHSA suicide prevention grant, and an NIH Disparity Center grant. CRCBH is now the agency that manages the SBHC for the Mescalero School.

Regular communication is key. As the national telehealth program quickly expanded, Dr. Fore and Dr. Bonham realized the importance of consistent communication. By scheduling a consistent, 30-min phone call each week, they are able to keep each other apprised of any changes or developments at any of the sites or within their respective systems. This regular communication helps them ensure that they are providing the same information to their partners and colleagues and to plan ahead for future growth.

Future Directions

The development of this initiative has had an interesting arc with some natural ups and downs. At any point, we could have decided that it was not working and let things dwindle away. Initially, there was a huge reliance on local champions such as Joe Glass and our first regional partners in the Nashville Area. Interestingly, when the clinical services were first developed, sites were offered free telepsychiatry services and there was very little response. Now, as telehealth services are becoming more common and providers hear from each other that there is value and benefit to setting up these services, TBHCE continues to receive more requests to start new clinical programs.

IHS and UNM worked together for over a year to develop a contract that allowed the partnership between two large institutions. This kind of contract was new for both systems and was not easy to negoti-

> *"The current collaboration has resulted from a perfect storm of relationships and timing."*

ate. The process of developing the contract was symbolic of the partnership, which involved a large amount of work, but all partners persisted with respectful communications because we felt that the effort was worthwhile. Similarly, the complicated credentialing process for clinical providers has also reflected everyone's commitment to the collaboration. Now we are at the stage when we are developing the first shared clinical position between the IHS and a university. The current collaboration has resulted from a perfect storm of relationships and timing.

References

1. Castor ML, Smyser MS, Taualii MM, Park AN, Lawson SA, Forquera RA et al. A nationwide population-based study identifying health disparities between American Indians/Alaska Natives and the general populations living in select urban counties. Am J Public Health. 2006;96:1478–84.
2. Gone J. Mental health services for Native Americans in the 21st century United States. Prof Psychol Res Pract. 2004;35:10–8.
3. Substance Abuse and Mental Health Services Administration. Results from the 2011 National Survey on Drug Use and Health, NSDUH Series H-45, HHS Publication No. (SMA) 12-4725. Rockville, MD: Substance Abuse and Mental Health Services Administration, 2012.
4. Herne MA, Bartholomew ML, Weahkee RL. Suicide mortality among American Indians and Alaska Natives, 1999–2009. Am J Public Health. 2014;104 Suppl 3:S336–42.
5. Mackin J, Perkins T, Furrer C. The power of protection: a population-based comparison of native and non-native youth suicide attempters. Am Indian Alsk Native Ment Health Res. 2012;19:20–54.
6. UNM School of Medicine Department of Psychiatry and Behavioral Sciences. Residency Opportunities: Rural. Available at http://psychiatry.unm.edu/education/residency/opportunities/Rural.html. Last accessed 23 Feb 2015.
7. Pew Research Center. 2012 American Community Survey. Available at http://www.pewresearch.org/fact-tank/2014/06/13/1-in-4-native-americans-and-alaska-natives-are-living-in-poverty/. Accessed 25 Oct 2014.

Narrative 7

The Program of Assertive Community Treatment and the University of Wisconsin Psychiatry Residency

John Battaglia, Art Walaszek, and Claudia L. Reardon

This is a story of an academic-community collaboration to create new educational experiences and models of team-based case management in the Program of Assertive Community Treatment in Madison, Wisconsin.

Central Moment

On July 21, 2010, Art Walaszek wrote to John Battaglia:

> Just a heads up … I'm going to have a preliminary discussion with the Associate Dean on Friday regarding University of Wisconsin Hospital and Clinics funding a PACT rotation. My initial proposal will be to fund one PGY4 resident for one day per week for a year (0.2 FTE). This would be part of a broader Community Psychiatry track within the PGY4 year.

Dr. Battaglia and Dr. Walaszek had formed a friendship while working together over several years on an inpatient psychiatry unit affiliated with the University of Wisconsin School of Medicine and Public Health (UW). Dr. Battaglia later left UW to become the psychiatrist at the Program of Assertive Community Treatment (PACT) in Madison, Wisconsin, and although PACT had no formal relationship with UW, he remained on as Adjunct Clinical Associate Professor of Psychiatry.

J. Battaglia, M.D. (✉) • A. Walaszek, M.D. • C.L. Reardon, M.D.
Department of Psychiatry, University of Wisconsin School of Medicine
and Public Health, Madison, WI, USA
e-mail: john.battaglia@dhs.wisconsin.gov; awalaszek@wisc.edu; clreardon@wisc.edu

© Springer International Publishing Switzerland 2015
L.W. Roberts et al. (eds.), *Partnerships for Mental Health*,
DOI 10.1007/978-3-319-18884-3_7

PACT is where it all began…the world's first psychiatric assertive community treatment. Sometimes referred to as "the Madison Model," PACT won the prestigious American Psychiatric Association 1974 Gold Achievement Award for innovation and excellence in community mental health [1]. PACT services include direct assistance with self-care skills, activities of daily living, housing, physical health care needs, vocational rehabilitation, educational rehabilitation, social skills training, AODA counseling, family counseling, supportive psychotherapy, cognitive behavioral therapy, medication monitoring, and intensive psychiatric treatment. In 1998 the National Alliance on Mental Illness (NAMI) recognized 25 years of the documented treatment success of the PACT model in serving people with severe mental illness and announced an initiative to bring the PACT treatment model to every state by 2002 [2]. At this time, PACT remains the gold standard for team-based, case management in the community for those suffering from chronic and severe mental illness.

Over four decades of existence, PACT has been a training site for assertive community treatment programs both within and outside the US. PACT has been a popular training site for social work interns, psychology interns, nursing students (including nurse practitioners), and occupational therapy students. Despite this rich heritage in community psychiatry training, PACT had not served as an educational resource for medical students or psychiatry residents at UW.

After Dr. Battaglia moved to PACT, Dr. Walaszek became the UW Psychiatry Residency Training Director. Claudia Reardon, M.D., was a resident in the training program under Dr. Walaszek's directorship. While a resident, she also met Dr. Battaglia, who, as an adjunct faculty member, served as her individual weekly supervisor and also presented seminars to her residency class. Through their continued professional and personal relationships, Drs. Battaglia, Walaszek, and Reardon realized the tremendous educational resource of PACT for students and residents at UW. Dr. Walaszek's message to Dr. Battaglia was the signal that, after years of discussion, a UW-PACT collaboration might finally happen.

One Partner's Story: John Battaglia

In my opinion, I am the luckiest psychiatrist in the world. In 2005 I was hired to be the psychiatrist for PACT in Madison, the Tigris and Euphrates Valley of assertive community treatment. This position was held formally for the most part by only one psychiatrist since the program began in the 1970s. It is, simply put, my dream job. I get to utilize all my skills and training in psychotherapy, crisis intervention, emergency psychiatry, psychopharmacology, and internal medicine for patients with severe and chronic mental illness, all of whom have failed to respond to the regular array of mental health services. I'm constantly stretching my psychopharmacology skills by utilizing novel, off label, and controversial treatments, because most PACT patients are treatment resistant to standard medication regimens. I'm the PACT team leader and I'm mobile, seeing patients wherever they need to be seen, whether at the PACT office, at their apartments, in group homes, at shelters, in the jail, or on the streets. This treatment mobility, while taxing at times, lends an essence of adventure and excitement to my work. With my PACT patients I have gone to picnics, been to the movies, celebrated holidays, attended high school graduations, and have also attended a wedding (of a PACT patient). Talk about being a multidimensional healer in all the best ways—I'm very involved in the lives of the most disadvantaged people on earth…and…I'm able to make a difference. Because of this high level of involvement, being a PACT psychiatrist involves a different level of responsibility for the PACT patients, a sense of "ownership" for the quality of their lives. PACT works, and I'm excited to be a part of it.

Since leaving full-time work at the UW in 2004, I've continued in my role as Adjunct Clinical Associate Professor through teaching seminars in community psychiatry and supportive psychotherapy and supervising residents. Always in the back of my mind was how to bring the educational gold mine of PACT to psychiatric trainees. Since it was established, PACT has been a substantial training program for students of all types as well as for mental health professionals from within and outside the US. The country of South Korea is currently embarking on a nationwide effort to incorporate the PACT model in all of its outpatient mental health clinics and has sent delegations of psychiatrists, nurses, social workers, and administrators to Madison PACT over the past decade for training. On a daily basis PACT staff are providing training for multiple levels of mental health trainees and professionals locally, regionally, and nationally. We live and breathe the PACT model and help others to do the same. The PACT esprit de corps is robust. There had to be a way to get this to UW psychiatric trainees.

One Partner's Story: Art Walaszek

In 2004, I was given a tremendous opportunity: to lead the UW Psychiatry Residency as it moved into a new world of Accreditation Council for Graduate Medical Education (ACGME) competencies and duty hours. Our residency's vision is "Psychiatry residents at the University of Wisconsin will compassionately and effectively care for the mental health of individuals and of the community, and will contribute to the field of medicine and to society through scholarship and service." This is a program with a rich tradition of community psychiatry training, with leaders in the field such as Len Stein and Ron Diamond involved in educating our residents for many years, and with clinical rotations at the Mental Health Center of Dane County (now Journey Mental Health Center). We also subscribe to the Wisconsin Idea, "the principle that the university should improve people's lives beyond the classroom … [through] teaching, research, outreach and public service" [3]. Thus, a critical goal for me has been to ensure that our residents have excellent training in community psychiatry. At the same time, I wanted to ensure that our residents were graduating truly prepared to practice twenty-first-century psychiatry, including being skilled at delivering evidence-based pharmacotherapy and psychotherapy; incorporating neuroscience into clinical practice; understanding the mental health system, and the role of psychiatrists in effecting change in that system; advocating for patients, including working with legislators and policy makers; providing care for an increasingly diverse population of patients; using the principles of quality improvement to continually enhance the care we provide; and working with our colleagues in primary care to deliver mental health care to large populations.

So, we faced a challenge: how do we expose residents to traditional community psychiatry models such as practiced at PACT (where our residents had not yet rotated) while simultaneously preparing them for new models of practice? We faced another challenge: how do we fund such educational experiences at a time of shrinking resources? My early discussions with Dr. Battaglia about a resident rotation at PACT had been hypothetical because I could not figure out a way to fund such a rotation. Though grant funding might have been available, it would not have resulted in sustained funding.

> *"So, we faced a challenge: how do we expose residents to traditional community psychiatry models such as practiced at PACT (where our residents had not yet rotated) while simultaneously preparing them for new models of practice? We faced another challenge: how do we fund such educational experiences at a time of shrinking resources?"*

An opportunity emerged in 2010. Six years into my role as residency training director, I had forged good relationships with the graduate medical education leadership at UW and had helped demonstrate the value of the residency to the institution. I argued that in order to continue to recruit outstanding residents to Madison, we had to demonstrate what was unique about us—and one way Madison distinguishes itself is by being the home of the agency that developed the ACT model. Offering a UW-funded rotation at PACT would help draw residents to Madison and would also help UW provide service to the community. Our Associate Dean (who oversees graduate medical education) agreed, and the UW Psychiatry Residency Community Psychiatry Track was born.

One Partner's Story: Claudia Reardon

In 2002, about 2 years before Dr. Battaglia would become the PACT psychiatrist and Dr. Walaszek would become the psychiatry residency training director, I (Claudia Reardon) was a first-year medical student at UW and started volunteering for a free psychiatry clinic housed in a shelter for homeless, seriously mentally ill people in Madison. I quickly came to love community psychiatry. Of all the patients with whom I interacted during medical school, those mentally ill patients in community settings inspired the most empathy in me, and they also seemed incredibly grateful for any care we were able to offer, even when it did not seem like much. At that time, I aspired to be a community psychiatrist.

During the next step on my educational journey, psychiatry residency at UW under Dr. Walaszek's leadership, I came to love what some would view as quite the opposite setting: academia. When the opportunity to take a UW faculty position as Associate Residency Program Director arose, I could not turn it down, because teaching and especially mentoring are among my favorite professional activities. With my appreciation for community psychiatry ongoing, it was important to me that residents in our program would be given opportunities to participate in "the Madison model" of care. It would be truly unfortunate if the psychiatry residency program in Madison could not offer training in this model! As a resident, I had traveled to the PACT building for my weekly supervision with Dr. Battaglia, and the atmosphere there always seemed so collegial and relaxed (some mental health providers even wore shorts during the summer—not something I was accustomed to seeing in the academic world). I have pleasant memories of sitting in the PACT waiting room alongside PACT clients as we exchanged conversational pleasantries, waiting for Dr. Battaglia to start our supervisory hour. Often such conversations were steeped in delusional thinking on the part of the clients, but regardless, they appeared to feel safe and cared for in the PACT environment. I wanted our residents to have the unique opportunity to rotate in the PACT setting, but unfortunately, challenges related to funding of community-based rotations for residents were increasing.

At the same time that Dr. Walaszek and I were interested in developing PACT opportunities for our residents, I also was reflecting on some of the most meaningful community-based mental health and public health experiences that I had had as a medical student and resident. Many of these were "by accident" experiences that various mentors or supervisors just happened to share with me, and they certainly had not come neatly packaged as a single rotation. It was only through ongoing experiences and interest in community and public health that big-picture themes such as the importance of advocacy for mentally ill patients became clear to me. I found myself wanting to create a "best of public health and psychiatry" elective, consisting of many of these experiences, for medical students who were interested in working with the poor, underserved, mentally ill in our community and who wanted to advocate for them on the systems level. It seemed that PACT would be an ideal core part of that type of experience. Moreover, it would provide an opportunity for any residents we would be able to have at PACT to interact with medical students with similar community-based interests. Our medical students continuously tell us how much they enjoy working with our residents, who are closer to their level developmentally and educationally.

Partners

After leaving our roles on the inpatient psychiatry unit affiliated with UW, we (Dr. Battaglia and Dr. Walaszek) continued to meet over the next several years. When Dr. Reardon arrived as a new faculty member, she joined in the discussions. The conversation of getting UW psychiatric trainees to PACT continued, sometimes directly with concomitant planning and strategizing. We were excited to make this happen, and conversations always had a synergistic mood with good alignment of our goals. The premier obstacle was funding; PACT is a state agency and no funding stream existed for trainees within the PACT budget (all current PACT trainees are funded by their respective training programs and agencies).

Dr. Battaglia met with PACT administrative staff to discuss the possibility of working with the UW psychiatry residency and received enthusiastic response. PACT already had in place a "culture of learning" with health care trainees in constant attendance at PACT as their primary clinical site. These ongoing academic partnerships include graduate level students in rehabilitation psychology, social work, and occupational therapy enrolled at UW, Madison College, and the University of Iowa. Twice PACT had accepted an advanced psychiatric nurse practitioner from UW for yearlong clinical internships under the direct supervision of Dr. Battaglia with good success. Also, part of the esprit de corps of PACT is to promote a culture of sensitivity and awareness for health care providers serving those with severe, chronic mental illness. PACT administrative staff viewed having direct influence on the training of UW psychiatry residents as a positive move, with an overall net benefit for people with severe mental illness.

A number of changes related to the structure and funding of rotations in the UW Psychiatry Residency led to new opportunities. First, Access Community Health Centers, a federally qualified health center, sought to partner with UW Health in the provision of mental health services. Access Community Health Centers provide medical, dental, and mental health care to a very underserved population; 48 % of their patients have Medicaid and 36 % were uninsured in 2012. Access started a psychiatric consultation service in 2007, and UW psychiatry residents began rotating there in 2010, learning a model of integrated care and psychiatric consultation to primary care in a community setting. The UW Hospital and Clinics, our residency's sponsoring institution, has funded the Access Community Health Centers rotation, consistent with its mission to partner with organizations in the community to provide better care for the people of our region. This rotation has become part of the core community psychiatry experience for all of our residents. Our colleagues, along with Dr. Reardon, have described this model in detail elsewhere [4].

Second, as mentioned earlier, Drs. Walaszek and Reardon recognized the need to continue to offer training in assertive community treatment. To that end, the UW Psychiatry Residency decided to develop a community psychiatry track to allow one to two residents per year to pursue specialized training in this model. Dr. Reardon took the lead in developing this track, as detailed elsewhere [5]. A critical issue was funding for this rotation, and in 2010, UW Hospitals and Clinics agreed to fund a pilot project that would cover each resident's stipend while on the rotation— specifically, one resident per year for one day per week throughout the year at the Madison PACT. An elective at an assertive community treatment team at the William S. Middleton VA Hospital, our VA partner, was already in place—the Madison PACT would become the site for a second community psychiatry resident.

Beginnings

PACT and the UW Psychiatry Residency Community Track

In October 2010, our residency education committee approved the addition of a community psychiatry track, with a goal of helping residents to:

- Acquire clinical expertise in caring for the seriously and persistently mentally ill in the community.
- Gain a comprehensive appreciation of the challenges, including those relating to social functioning, physical and psychiatric health, and day-to-day community functioning, faced by the severely and persistently mentally ill.
- Develop an understanding of the importance of and skill in serving as a member of an interdisciplinary team in caring for the seriously and persistently mentally ill.

We promoted the new track to our third-year residents and sought applications from them for the 2011–2012 academic year. We also indicated to our residency applicants that year (and since then) that we had developed the community psychiatry track. Our application process has involved asking residents what they would like to accomplish by participating in the track, how they envision their participation in this track impacting their career, and whether they appreciate the role of a psychiatrist within an interdisciplinary community psychiatry team. Passion for working for people with severe, persistent mental illness and willingness to immerse oneself in the team are critical. We named our first community psychiatry track resident in December 2010, and the clinical experience at PACT began in July 2011.

UW Medical Student Psychiatry Elective in Public Health

In 2011, the UW School of Medicine and Public Health put forth a call to its respective departments for development of electives with a public health theme for fourth-year medical students. Accordingly, Dr. Reardon worked with a number of community resources to develop a proposal for such an elective, titled "Public health advocacy and service in psychiatry." The proposal was approved and garnered grant money from the medical school to develop the elective, which was offered to medical students beginning in July 2012.

Specific learning objectives developed for the elective were that, by the end of the rotation, students should be able to:

- Discuss the role of socioeconomic, environmental, and cultural determinants of health on the mental health status and mental health care of individuals and populations.
- Design and record a public service announcement on a psychiatric public health issue.

- Appraise the quality of the evidence of peer-reviewed medical and public health literature in developing a brief presentation on a specific topic related to preventive or public health care in psychiatry.
- List and describe a variety of community resources available to improve the mental health of individuals and populations, especially those that are underserved.
- Engage effectively with legislators and/or members of professional medical advocacy organizations in discussing psychiatric public health issues.

Interventions

UW Psychiatry Residency Community Track

The fourth-year psychiatry resident in the UW community psychiatry track is assigned to PACT for a 20 % position. The initial part of the training at PACT involved shadowing Dr. Battaglia and various PACT staff during clinical encounters, group therapies, and daily morning report (similar to inpatient multidisciplinary staff rounds). Because the fourth-year resident is in a relatively advanced stage of psychiatric training, taking such a passive role initially required some shifting of cognitive set (watch rather than do). Once the shift was made, however, the PACT psychiatry residents have enjoyed the process of doing such unusual work, for example, accompanying a patient for grocery shopping or taking a patient to a medical appointment. PACT has a unique patient population of severe, treatment resistant mentally ill who have failed to thrive in the usual community treatment array of psychiatric services. Many patients are undergoing off-label and combination pharmacologic regimens with which the psychiatry residents have no prior experience. For this reason, the residents are assigned to clinical care of just a few patients during the PACT elective. This allows for Dr. Battaglia to comprehensively supervise each case, especially with psychopharmacology management. At least once they are assigned to an intake of a new PACT referral, in order to learn the PACT evaluation and initial treatment planning process. They then continue to provide care for this patient throughout the remaining year of their PACT experience. Once the PACT resident is familiar with PACT multidisciplinary treatment and procedures, he or she begins seeing PACT patients in community settings.

Each PACT psychiatry resident undergoes relatively extensive supervision from Dr. Battaglia, including supervision of encounters in real time (both in the PACT office and in the community). This level of supervision, watching the resident interact clinically with a patient and providing immediate feedback, is a remarkably rich learning opportunity for the PACT psychiatry resident. The residents are also coached on becoming an effective PACT treatment team member, both in medical leadership and in learning to recognize and utilize the contributions of each team member. Each PACT resident has also developed her or his own niche for helping the multidisciplinary team. For example, one resident helped with development of a PACT social skills group, and another developed a group experience for PACT trainees/new hires for coping with the stress of working in the intense case management format at PACT.

Several challenges have emerged for the PACT psychiatry resident. The biggest challenge has been keeping the resident current with the patients' clinical condition while working only 20 % time (two half days weekly). The PACT unit runs much like an inpatient psychiatry unit, with daily rounds and need at times for daily treatment changes. Although the resident is updated at the beginning of the work shift, there remains significant information sharing, planning, and treatment decisions that occur in the resident's absence. Also, a key "value" in PACT psychiatry work comes from being consistently available and taking responsibility in the continuum of care for patients with severe and chronic mental illness. The PACT psychiatrist often provides non-psychiatric medical evaluation and treatment. As described previously, this "ownership" is an important value of the PACT psychiatrist identity. PACT is a 24-hour service agency, and patients often view their PACT providers as stable and available, regardless of circumstance. This concept of the need for the PACT psychiatrists to be available to their patients has sometimes been challenged by absence of the psychiatry resident for the majority of the time. Some PACT patients have expressed the feeling that they are getting less comprehensive or less advanced psychiatric care from the PACT resident, based some on the "part-time" presence. Supervision of the PACT resident has included review of the concept of responsibility, with particular attention to professional identity. For a PACT psychiatrist the notion of ownership goes beyond the idea of "shift work" to providing comprehensive care despite what are assumed to be regular work shifts. Residents are encouraged to be flexible and creative to provide comprehensive care regardless of the 20 % on-site time constraints.

A PACT community psychiatry resident was assigned to a 52-year-old woman with treatment-resistant schizophrenia, residing in a community-based facility. The patient had severe and chronic auditory hallucinations, persecutory delusions, labile mood, and disorganization (often unable to state her name or birth date). She was severely symptomatic despite robust treatment with multiple antipsychotic medications, mood stabilizers, and augmentation with off-label medication approaches. The PACT resident saw the patient weekly at her residential facility and coordinated with the PACT treatment team and staff at the residence. She determined a trial of fish oil capsules was indicated from her evidence-based review of treatment-resistant schizophrenia and the history of past failed treatment attempts. She underwent training on the use of the Brief Psychiatric Rating Scale and began weekly ratings on the patient during a clinical trial of fish oil capsules. The patient showed mild improvement in disorganization, mood lability, and hallucinatory behavior. Her improvement allowed her to start a part-time job assembling business fliers at the PACT office.

Beyond the PACT experience, the community psychiatry track residents have a wealth of other experiences to enrich their community psychiatry training [5]. They are encouraged to serve regularly at a volunteer psychiatry clinic in Madison for the homeless, seriously mentally ill of the city. They present a community psychiatry seminar on a topic of their choosing as a "guest lecturer" for the third-year residents' community psychiatry seminar series. Additionally, they present a teleconference on a community psychiatry topic of their choice as part of the Wisconsin Public Psychiatry Network Conference Series. We encourage them to attend the Institute on Psychiatric Services national meeting and to submit a poster or workshop abstract for that meeting on a community psychiatry-related topic. They may also attend a NAMI Wisconsin Board of Directors meeting (Dr. Battaglia serves on this board). Finally, they choose a community psychiatry track mentor, who meets with them regularly and helps to put their community psychiatry experiences into perspective.

UW Medical Student Psychiatry Elective in Public Health

The "public health advocacy and service in psychiatry" elective offers experiences in two main areas of public health: public health service and public health advocacy. Within the area of public health service, a core feature is time at PACT. Additionally, the students spend time within two different mental health integrated care settings: Access Community Health Centers and the VA Integrated Care Clinic. The students are also exposed to the clubhouse model of community mental health treatment. Within the area of public health advocacy, students work with the Wisconsin Medical Society to record a public service announcement on a psychiatry public health issue. The students have hands-on advocacy experience by going with the Wisconsin Medical Society government relations staff to the Wisconsin State Capitol to advocate on any of a number of timely mental health issues. Students attend any legislative council or board meetings of the Wisconsin Medical Society or Dane County Medical Society that happen during the time of their elective. Finally, the students write a blog on a psychiatry public health issue, and after review and editing by Dr. Reardon, it is posted on the American Psychiatric Association's Healthy Minds website, for which Dr. Reardon is a blogger. The students meet regularly with Dr. Reardon to reflect on their elective experiences.

Outcomes

PACT and the Community Psychiatry Track

Since the inception of the community psychiatry track in the 2011–2012 academic year, we have trained three residents, with a fourth currently in training. Our first graduate completed an addiction psychiatry fellowship and now practices at a non-profit mental health and addictions treatment center. Our second graduate practices psychiatry in the VA system after completing a forensic psychiatry fellowship. Our third track member is in a community psychiatry fellowship. Anecdotally, our being able to offer the community psychiatry track has seemed to help with our residency recruitment efforts. For example, our fourth community psychiatry track member states that the reason she chose our residency program is because of that track.

The residents have well received the PACT clinical experience. The residents' average rating of the rotation has been 5 ("outstanding" on a five-point Likert scale) in considering how satisfied they were with the rotation. Representative resident comments on evaluation forms have included the following:

> *"Really wish more people could experience what this rotation is like. It is amazing how supportive, caring, and enthusiastic staff are to really provide care."*
> *"This rotation is amazing! The staff are wonderful and accepting of [residents]. It is nice to be actively included as a member of the treatment team within a matter of a couple of weeks."*
> *"Fills a great need in the training program. Highly recommend to other residents interested in seeing chronic treatment-resistant psychotic illness up close in Madison."*

As mentioned, community psychiatry residents are also encouraged to participate in scholarly activities such as presentations of posters, workshops, and teleconferences at state and national meetings. Scholarly outcomes related to community psychiatry for our three residents who have gone through the track thus far include one national workshop, five national posters, two statewide teleconferences, one presentation at the NAMI Wisconsin Annual Conference, and two articles for the NAMI Wisconsin newsletter.

Comments from past community psychiatry track residents:

> *"I feel like I am contributing to people's lives in a more intimate and more meaningful way. Getting to know people on a different level than you get in regular outpatient is far more satisfying for me. It is a good personality fit for me. I would rather talk with someone about their voices—the experiences of it, the perception of it, how to cope with it—than about other types of symptoms."*
> *"I feel like I have had very solid training in this patient population, working with a team, looking at group dynamics, and could easily step into a team for a community mental health center. I opted for more training (fellowship in community psychiatry), which will facilitate being able to be more of a leader on that team."*

Medical Student Elective

Eight students have taken the medical student elective over the 2 years that it has been offered. All the students have rated the elective as a 5 ("strongly agree" on a five-point Likert scale) in considering if the elective provided adequate opportunities to understand the intersection between public health and individual patient care; if the elective allowed them to see how they could integrate its public health content into their future practice; and overall, if the elective provided a good learning experience. Qualitatively, student evaluation comments are represented by the following quote:

> *"This was a fantastic rotation for individuals not only interested in psychiatry. Having a solid grasp on the mental health options for patients is something that anyone entering primary care should be aware of. It was exciting to go to a different environment each day.*

I almost felt like I wasn't a medical student as some of the models push you to expand upon your previous perceived boundaries. The contact people at each site were welcoming and enthusiastic to incorporate me into their day. At the end of the week, debriefing with Dr. Reardon allowed me to process everything I was witnessing. It is an infectious atmosphere and one in which I thoroughly enjoyed myself. Oh yeah, I also learned a ton!"

We believe that this elective has allowed us to reestablish the residency's reputation among UW medical students interested in psychiatry as an excellent place to learn community psychiatry. Two of our three fourth-year UW medical students who took the elective within the past year matched into our program for their upcoming psychiatry residency training.

Conclusion

Assertive community treatment was initially developed in Madison, Wisconsin, and remains a gold standard for treatment of people with serious and chronic mental illness. Declining funding and other issues has resulted in challenges with providing community psychiatry training for residents. Developing a community psychiatry track for fourth-year residents with a core clinical experience at the Madison Program of Assertive Community Treatment has resulted in improved community psychiatry training and has spurred educational developments for medical students with an interest in public mental health.

References

1. American Psychiatric Association Gold Award: A community treatment program. Mendota Mental Health Institute, Madison, Wisconsin. Hospital and Community Psychiatry. 1974;25:669–72.
2. Assertive Community Treatment. National Alliance on Mental Illness. Available at https://www.nami.org/Template.cfm?Section=ACT-TA_Center&template=/ContentManagement/ContentDisplay.cfm&ContentID=33331. Last accessed 1 Apr 2014.
3. The Wisconsin Idea: Advancing health and medicine. University of Wisconsin-Madison.. Available at http://www.wisconsinidea.wisc.edu/get-involved/. Last accessed 1 Apr 2014.
4. Zeidler Schreiter EA, Pandhi N, Fondwo MD, Thomas C, Vonk J, Reardon CL, et al. Consulting psychiatry within an integrated primary care model. J Health Care Poor Underserved. 2013;24:1522–30.
5. Reardon CL, Factor RM, Brenner CJ, Singh P, Spurgeon JA. Community psychiatry tracks for residents: a review of four programs. Community Ment Health J. 2014;50:10–6.

Narrative 8
Laughing at the Rain

Daryn Reicherter

This is a story of how physicians worked together with a local residential program for homeless and marginally housed people in Palo Alto, California, providing care for people of the streets, the parks, and the shelters.

We had finished the mental health questionnaire, but the man I had interviewed could not get up from the street corner where we sat. His uncontrolled diabetes overwhelmed him. "Gotta eat," he said. "Can I just sit a while here and eat? Then I'll be on my way," his gaunt face asked while his thin fingers fumbled through his bag for a cup-of-soup. His breaths gasped, exhausted by the effort. His eyes surveyed the street then found mine for an answer to his request.

"Please, stay and eat."

He was sick. He was homeless. It looked like it might start raining.

In preparation for the opening of a local residential program for homeless and marginally housed people, my colleague and I had been conducting mental health interviews for Palo Alto's unhoused population. The process for selecting candidates to become residents at the new center was underway. We interviewed candidates over a 4-month period. We met more than 200 individuals from the San Francisco's mid-peninsula, each with a unique and often tragic story. Each story broke all expectations of how people become homeless. We met unemployed computer engineers living in their cars. We met political refugees unable to translate

D. Reicherter, M.D. (✉)
Department of Psychiatry and Behavioral Sciences, Stanford University School of Medicine, Stanford, CA, USA
e-mail: reichertermd@yahoo.com

© Springer International Publishing Switzerland 2015
L.W. Roberts et al. (eds.), *Partnerships for Mental Health*,
DOI 10.1007/978-3-319-18884-3_8

their professional skills into US licensing standards. We met single mothers with children fighting for a place to sleep in the shelter system. We met severely mentally ill persons who had never been picked up by the state's welfare system.

We met them on the streets, in the parks, at the homeless drop-in center, and in the shelters.

"Never thought I'd end up like this," the man said after his soup had given him enough energy to sit upright. He talked awhile about his experience of homelessness. He told me about nights by the creek, under the bridge with that cold, mocking rain oppressing his very movement. He told me about lost pride and having to stand at a stoplight with a cardboard sign asking strangers for money. He told me about how his failing health and advancing age made the struggle against the elements more doubtful.

"And all winter long, that rain, laughin' at me." His teeth clenched. His eyes narrowed. "Just *laughin'* at me."

Down the street, construction commenced on the new homeless center. The project was, at that time, just weeks from completion. Eighteen rooms for families adjoined 70 single occupancy rooms that were built and were getting their "final touches" while the homeless people eagerly waited. The housing units rose above a first-floor service area that would be devoted to essential services including social work, medical, and mental health. All services would be included in one center with the intention of transitioning unhoused individuals from homelessness to permanent housing.

But to create and sustain such an immense community project requires *partnerships* between invested individuals, programs, and potential clients. The story of the partnerships in instances like this one is often never told. Occasionally, heartwarming outcomes might be reported in the local newspapers—or, rarely, in professional journals. The opening day ribbon-cutting ceremony might be a local news feature. But the struggle and commitment of the *partners* is often an untold story. It takes planning, effort, and deep and abiding collaboration to get a program in place to help a homeless man get out of the rain.

He sighed, still too weak to get to his feet, then continued. "I guess I give the rain something to laugh at." His hand gesture alluded to his body's weakness. He had been a great athlete in his youth. He had worked hard, physical jobs most of his life. And he could not pinpoint any event or circumstance that had led to his current situation. He never had a problem with alcohol or drugs. He never had problems with the law. But as problems developed with his health so did they develop with his

> "...to create and sustain such an immense community project requires partnerships between invested individuals, programs, and potential clients. The story of the partnerships in instances like this one is often never told. Occasionally, heartwarming outcomes might be reported in the local newspapers – or, rarely, in professional journals. The opening day ribbon-cutting ceremony might be a local news feature. But the struggle and commitment of the partners is often and untold story. It takes planning, effort, and deep and abiding collaboration to get a program in place to help a homeless man get out of the rain."

economic state. Fading health seemed to accompany him on his path to his daily interface with the sun, the wind, and the rain—the mocking rain.

The local center was the culmination of inspiring ideas and tireless efforts and great collaboration—true partnerships among diverse (and maybe even unlikely) colleagues, working together with a common goal. Years in the making, with heroic, aspirational, and sometimes comical stories of how the partners strategized, sacrificed, and even sparred with each other to establish the community resource.

After we talked a long while, my conversation partner strained to rise and straightened his hat. His bag of belongings swung over his shoulder, he paused before starting back to his stoplight with his cardboard sign.

"A man my age shouldn't be living like this." He had told me that he did not want to let his hopes get too high about getting housing at the center. He was accustomed to disappointment.

"But I would like to be inside when that rain starts coming to laugh at me again." He stared straight ahead with a stiff smile on his face as though he could see what he was saying while the words came out.

"Then I could be laughin' at that rain instead of that rain laughin' at me."

The Opportunity Center of the mid-peninsula had its official ribbon-cutting ceremony on September 17, 2005. Eighteen families and 70 single people moved from the street into housing, and services were opened to homeless persons from the area. The outcomes were published in medical and social work journals. The opening gala was in the local news. But the partnerships that laid the foundation for those outcomes never received particular attention. The successes and failures of the process were not articulated or documented, so they cannot serve as a lighthouse for similar projects to follow. This narrative shines light on the process of academic-community partnerships that have brought about novel resources to address needs and fulfill goals of mutual importance—even if the goal is simply getting a few people out of the rain.

Narrative 9
From the Ivory Tower to the Real World: Translating an Evidence-Based Intervention for Latino Dementia Family Caregivers into a Community Setting

Dolores Gallagher-Thompson, Paula Alvarez, Veronica Cardenas, Marian Tzuang, Roberto E. Velasquez, Kurt Buske, and Lorie Van Tilburg

This is the story of how academic researchers worked together with a community resource center to provide support for Latino caregivers of Alzheimer's disease patients, and improve quality of life for this underserved population.

Globally, the number of older adults is increasing substantially. According to the World Health Organization [1], by the year 2050 there will be two billion people over the age of 60 around the world. In the United States, Latinos are the

D. Gallagher-Thompson, Ph.D., A.B.P.P. (✉)
Department of Psychiatry and Behavioral Sciences, Stanford University School of Medicine, Stanford, CA, USA
e-mail: dolorest@stanford.edu

P. Alvarez, Ph.D.
Palo Alto University, Pacific Graduate School of Psychology, Palo Alto, CA, USA
e-mail: paula_alvarez@ymail.com

V. Cardenas, Ph.D.
Department of Psychiatry, University of California, San Diego, CA, USA
e-mail: vcardenas@ucsd.edu

M. Tzuang, M.S.W.
Stanford University School of Medicine, Stanford Geriatric Education Center, Stanford, CA, USA
e-mail: mtzuang@stanford.edu

R.E. Velasquez, M.S. • L. Van Tilburg, M.S.W.
Southern Caregiver Resource Center, San Diego, CA, USA
e-mail: RVelasquez@caregivercenter.org; LVanTilburg@caregivercenter.org

K. Buske, M.S.W.
Consultant
e-mail: kurtbuske@yahoo.com

© Springer International Publishing Switzerland 2015
L.W. Roberts et al. (eds.), *Partnerships for Mental Health*,
DOI 10.1007/978-3-319-18884-3_9

fastest-growing ethnic minority group. It has been estimated that older Latinos will represent 20 % of the US older population by 2050 [2]. As the average age of the population increases, the number of people developing Alzheimer's disease also increases. In the general population of older adults, the prevalence of major neuro-cognitive disorder (also known as dementia) due to Alzheimer's disease has been reported to be approximately 7 % for individuals between 65 and 74 years, 53 % for those between 75 and 84 years, and 40 % for individuals over the age of 85 years [3]. Although prevalence rates are similar, the absolute number of Latinos who suffer from Alzheimer's disease is expected to increase 600 % by 2050 due to increasing longevity and related factors [4]. According to Clark et al. [5], Latinos start experiencing symptoms of Alzheimer's disease approximately, on average, 7 years earlier than non-Hispanic Whites. Hinton et al. [6] describe a greater burden on Latino family caregivers due to higher prevalence of significant behavioral problems (e.g., hallucinations, aggression, wandering), suggesting that this group is in particular need of appropriate services.

According to the Alzheimer's Association [7], there are currently approximately 15 million unpaid caregivers in the US. In the year 2012, it was estimated that these caregivers provided over 17.5 billion hours of care [7]. Family members usually become the primary caregivers of their loved ones until the illness becomes so severe that they might seek out help in long-term care facilities such as nursing homes. In many ethnically diverse communities, however, such as those of Latino and Asian origins, family members do not see nursing homes as an acceptable alternative. Generally, the oldest daughter (or son) is expected to become the primary caregiver and remain in that role for the duration of the illness [6]. In their meta-analysis, Pinquart and Sörensen [8] found that Latino and Asian American caregivers were more depressed, provided more hands-on care, had stronger filial obligation beliefs, and reported poorer physical health than non-Hispanic Whites and others with whom they were compared. It has also been reported that caregivers' mortality rate may increase along with their stress and depression [9, 10].

Given the serious responsibilities and health risks that are associated with caring for a loved one with Alzheimer's disease, most caregivers would benefit from receiving information, emotional support, and skill training [11]. Many are not aware of how to obtain much needed help to decrease their levels of stress and improve their well-being, however. Latino caregivers also face other challenges, such as lack of English proficiency, financial constraints, negative stigma towards Alzheimer's disease, and limited formal education as well as a dearth of programs developed to meet their specific needs [12, 13].

To help decrease the existing mental health services disparity among Latinos, Dr. Gallagher-Thompson and her colleagues were key participants in an influential series of studies that included a large number of Latino caregivers of elders with dementia. The first study, Resources for Enhancing Alzheimer's Caregiver Health (REACH I), was a product of collaboration among six sites in the US that recruited dementia family caregivers from Birmingham, AL; Boston, MA; Memphis, TN; Miami, FL; Palo Alto, CA; and Philadelphia, PA. The primary purpose of these projects was to tailor interventions (unique to each site) to meet the specific needs of racially and ethnically diverse clients at these locations. Latino caregivers represent a key focus at the Palo Alto and Miami sites. At Miami, 225 (114 Cuban American and 111 White American) caregivers were randomized to (1) a family-therapy-based in-home intervention, (2) a combination of that intervention and a computer telephone integration system designed to augment it, or (3) a control condition where minimal contact and support such as active listening and written information about dementia and caregiving were given to caregivers over the phone. Caregivers who received the combined intervention saw a significant reduction in depressive symptoms at 6 months. This program was particularly beneficial for Cuban American husband and daughter caregivers over time (based on follow-up at 18-months) [14].

At Palo Alto, 122 Anglo and 91 Latino caregivers of elder relatives with dementia were randomly assigned to either a cognitive behavior therapy (CBT)—based "coping skills" psychoeducational program or to a support group control condition patterned after those available in the community. Those assigned to the control condition met weekly for 12 weeks to discuss challenges and receive support from one another. In contrast, those assigned to the intervention group were given a workbook and participated in 12 small group meetings that focused on skill training. Sessions were offered in Spanish or English as appropriate. Bilingual/bicultural interventionists led the Spanish language meetings.

Each group included six to ten caregivers as a way to increase social support from nonfamily members. During these sessions caregivers learned a variety of skills for mood and behavior management (e.g., how to relax during stressful caregiving moments and how to get help and support from family members by learning to communicate effectively and express their needs). Caregivers were also encouraged to engage in pleasant activities (small and positive activities for themselves daily), with the understanding that these behaviors would help improve their mood. Since the majority reported depressive symptoms, they were also encouraged to set self-change goals and reward themselves for any accomplishments. At the end of this program, both Latino and Anglo caregivers reported fewer depressive symptoms, better coping skills, better interactions with their social networks, and more tolerance toward their care-recipient's memory and behavioral problems than caregivers of either ethnicity in the control condition [15].

The second study, REACH II, enrolled from five of the original six sites a total of 642 dementia family caregivers: 212 were Latino, 219 were White/Caucasian, and 211 were Black/African American. Caregivers were randomly assigned, within each ethnic group, to either the control group, which consisted of minimal contact through follow-up phone calls, or the intervention group. The latter consisted of a combination of 12 behavior management-focused home visits and telephone-based support groups and discussion of the caregiver's physical health and well-being. Caregivers in the intervention group reported greater improvement on several quality-of-life indices from pre- to post-assessment measures than those in the control condition, irrespective of race/ethnicity. One of the most significant findings of this study was that Latinos showed the greatest improvement in comparison with the other two ethnic groups [16].

The Local Community

Around the same time the researchers of the REACH I project were publishing their findings and the REACH II project was under development, California was going through some exciting changes promising to improve public mental health services. In November 2004, Proposition 63, also known as the Mental Health Services Act (MHSA), was passed, and individuals making above one million dollars started being taxed an additional 1 % on their personal income [17]. This bill provided the first opportunity in many years to expand county mental health programs for individuals throughout different age groups, including older adults and families. The primary goal of Proposition 63 was to provide prevention, early intervention, and evidence-based treatments. Each county in California was expected to come up with a plan on how to address these new demands. Roberto Velasquez was working for the Alzheimer's Association San Diego Chapter at the time and was very aware of the high needs that Latino caregivers in that region were facing. Mr. Velasquez became part of the special community advising committee for San Diego County and realized the need for local services for Latino dementia caregivers.

To increase awareness of the need for services for dementia family caregivers among county leaders, Mr. Velasquez requested and obtained funding from the BRAVO foundation and collaborated with a team of researchers at San Diego State University (led by Drs. Ramon Valle and Mario D. Garrett) to investigate the prevalence of Alzheimer's disease and associated dementias among Latinos in San Diego County. The results of their investigation suggested that the Latino population over the age of 60 is projected to grow 344 % by 2030 and 652 % by 2050. Valle et al. [18] concluded that the number of Latino family members experiencing caregiving burden and stress is expected to rapidly increase to close to 100,000 individuals by the year of 2050. Thus, creating local services to provide intervention for caregivers is imperative.

With this new information, Mr. Velasquez developed a report for San Diego County leaders explaining the demographics associated with Alzheimer's disease and associated dementias and highlighting several other important issues. Latinos were at higher risk to develop cardiovascular diseases and diabetes, making them more vulnerable to develop Alzheimer's disease [19]. Latinos are the fastest-growing minority in that region, and they provide care at home for their loved ones as a way to prevent institutionalization [20]. One challenge was to clarify to county leaders that the proposed services were not meant to target the medical illness of dementia but to help the caregivers of persons with Alzheimer's disease with their stress and depression. A second challenge was to identify evidence-based treatments for Latino caregivers, given that this population has been understudied. After a thorough literature review, Mr. Velasquez identified the REACH studies as the most reasonable choice for the proposed county program.

Academia Meets Community

The Southern Caregiver Resource Center (SCRC) is an independent nonprofit agency founded in 1987 and based in southern San Diego County. In 2009, the Rosalynn Carter Institute for Caregiving awarded the SCRC a Quality Care Connections grant of $100,000 for 2 years to implement the REACH II program with Latino caregivers. The goal of this grant was to serve 25 caregivers annually with this intensive, home-based program. Mr. Velasquez's local advocacy efforts started to show results early in 2009, when San Diego County released a request for proposals to develop and implement services targeting Latino caregivers using one of the REACH models. Mr. Velasquez, who was by then working for the SCRC, asked Dr. Gallagher-Thompson, a principal investigator for the REACH projects, for help to write this proposal.

Dr. Gallagher-Thompson assisted Mr. Velasquez to shape the county proposal to meet the county's goal of 200 caregivers to complete the program within a 12-month period, which could not be done if the full REACH II protocol was followed. They selected the Spanish-language version of the REACH I small group program as the most appropriate intervention for the county proposal. In late October 2009, San Diego County awarded the contract to SCRC. Thus, the SCRC would offer both programs in parallel—one to fulfill the Rosalynn Carter funding initiative and the other, the San Diego County contract.

The Partnership

To help ensure the success of these programs and overcome cultural barriers, community partnerships were established first, with organizations that already provided health-related services to the Latino community. Evidence suggests that Latinos are more likely to enroll and stay in programs when recruited through a professional referral source that is well trusted [21]. The SCRC hired four *promotoras* from the local San Ysidro Health Center and the *La Maestra* Community Health Center who were trained on topics related to dementia and caregiving stress (in addition to their role as bilingual/bicultural health educators).

Promotoras (community peer educators/counselors or community health advocates) are essential to successful outreach in the Latino community. These trusted individuals, usually women, are friendly faces in the community that help provide information and education to families and are critical to generating referrals for the program intervention. They, an employee of the respected partner agencies, help instill *confianza* (trust) in the community about the program (Fig. 9.1).

The *La Maestra* Community Health Center and San Ysidro Health Center were selected as partners for this program for many reasons, such as their more than 75 years of providing exemplary health and mental health services to San Diego's Latino community, but equally important was the leadership of both these agencies. Mr. Velasquez had worked closely with the former chief executive officer of San

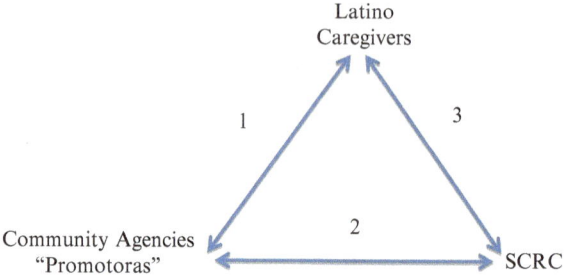

Fig. 9.1 "The Confianza Triangle" of successful recruitment as applied to the Southern Caregiver Resource Center (SCRC) example in this chapter. In the figure, (1) a community agency first establishes trust with Latino individuals, (2) the researcher (or SCRC) establishes trust with the community agency, and (3) the researcher (or SCRC) indirectly establishes trust with the Latino individuals

Ysidro Health Center, Mr. Ed Martinez, for over 10 years on Latino and dementia programs, which included the Dementia Care Network project (*El Portal de Esperanza,* "the Portal of Hope") developed by Mr. Velasquez in 2002 and funded by The California Endowment and a physician education project in 2003 funded by Forest Laboratories. Mr. Velasquez and Mr. Martinez engaged in collaborative programs educating families, professionals, and elected officials about the growing concern of Alzheimer's disease and associated dementias in the Latino community.

After an introduction by Mr. Martinez, Mr. Velasquez developed a relationship with Ms. Zara Marselian, chief executive officer for *La Maestra* Community Health Centers, who also began collaborating on dementia-specific projects with Mr. Velasquez and Mr. Martinez. After the Dementia Care Network project ended, Mr. Martinez and Ms. Marselian jointly funded a Memory Screening Clinic in collaboration with the University of California San Diego that continues to operate to this day. When San Diego County Behavioral Health Services and Rosalynn Carter Institute for Caregiving presented the opportunity to develop a REACH program in San Diego, Mr. Velasquez knew that both the San Ysidro Health Center and *La Maestra* Community Health Center would be a natural match for the program because of the commitment from their leadership.

After the partnerships were in place, a small team of external consultants was engaged to evaluate the SCRC's readiness and cultural competence to engage the Latino community effectively and deliver the evidence-based programs with fidelity to the original REACH protocols.

Next, an advisory committee was formed, consisting of several original REACH researchers, Latino dementia caregivers, local university professors, *promotoras* from partnering agencies, and the SCRC's management team. The committee met regularly to discuss ways to tailor the REACH protocols to fit the unique needs of Latino caregivers in San Diego County. The committee evaluated two proposed treatment modalities (and written materials that went with them) for their cultural relevance and sensitivity, clarity, and likely effectiveness with the target group. Special emphasis was made on certain components that these modified interventions needed to have to ensure fidelity to the original programs from which they derived.

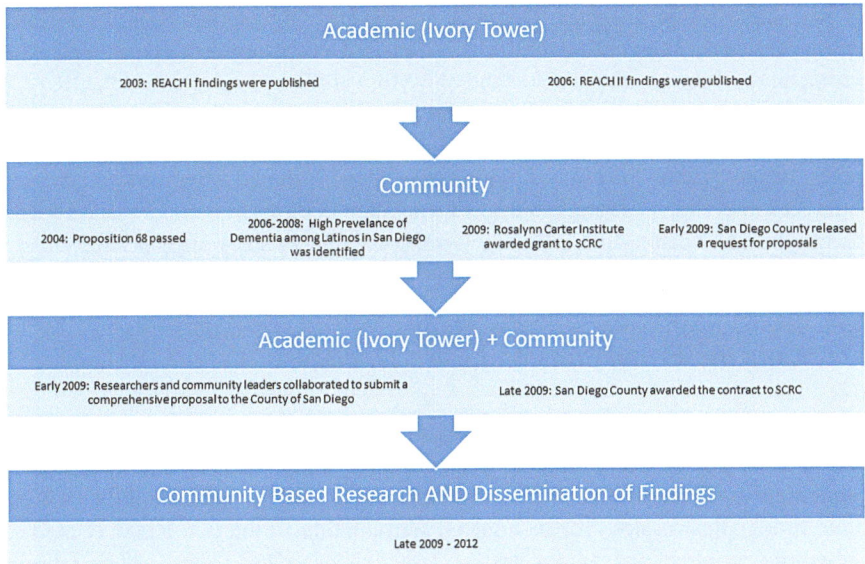

Fig. 9.2 Chronology of partnership

These components included keeping patients and caregivers safe; caregivers learning to manage (or respond differently) to difficult behaviors from the person with dementia; caregivers learning skills to handle negative emotions; and caregivers practicing a range of communication skills—especially how to obtain more help from other family members. Providing information on local resources was also critical. In addition, for practical reasons (e.g., staffing and overall costs), each of the original programs needed to be shortened.

Lastly, because data collection plays an important role in the evaluation of an evidence-based program, the SCRC partnered with the Health Services Research Center (HSRC) at University of California San Diego to develop a database to house the data obtained from the baseline and post-treatment assessments. The HSRC also provided technical assistance on data tracking and monitoring and prepared the empirical reports that were submitted back to funding sources.

Figure 9.2 depicts the chronology of how the partnership has formed and the actions taken to implement and evaluate the program.

Implementation: Examples of "Culturally Tailoring"

Renaming the Program

The acronym of the program, REACH, does not correspond to a word with any meaning in Spanish. Based on careful considerations from several focus groups consisting of dementia caregivers, *promotoras,* and care managers, we renamed REACH

I (the small group program) CALMA (*Cuidadores Acompañándose y Luchando para Mejorar y Seguir Adelante,* which translates to "caregivers giving each other company and striving to get better and move forward"), and we renamed the REACH II program (based on in-home visits and provision of extensive information about caregiving and cognitive impairment) CUIDAR (*Cuidadores Unidos Inspirados en Dar Amor y buscar Respuestas,* which translates to "united caregivers to give love and seek answers"). Although the new names are not direct or literal translations, the acronyms are meaningful to the target group and conceptually appropriate.

Training the Promotoras and Care Managers

Training workshops for *promotoras* orient them to the SCRC services and teach them about key aspects related to dementia caregiving. The original length of the training was 10 hours (five 2-hour sessions), but we later condensed it into 5 hours due to logistical issues. Topics covered introduction to the two REACH models, eligibility criteria, and administrative protocols/procedures (e.g., referral protocols); additional services available in the San Diego area for older adults and caregivers; elder abuse and mandated reporting laws; Alzheimer's disease, dementia, and related cultural beliefs (e.g., Alzheimer's disease being equal to normal aging); skills to reduce caregiver stress; and plans for monthly *promotora* meetings and regular in-services. Lastly, we gave *promotoras* reading materials in both English and Spanish on topics related to Alzheimer's disease and associated dementias, caregiving facts and statistics, and common signs of depression and anxiety.

The purpose of the 2-day training workshop for care managers was to train the two bilingual/bicultural master's degree-level care managers hired by the SCRC to deliver the REACH interventions. On the first day, Dr. Gallagher-Thompson and Dr. Cardenas trained them in how to deliver the CUIDAR home-based caregiver intervention (corresponding to REACH II). They highlighted adherence to the original treatment protocol by including topics such as the following:

- CBT (the theoretical base from which the program was developed)
- Identifying caregivers' risk priorities
- Simple relaxation techniques (e.g., breathing exercises)
- Using a "stress diary" to log stress and anxiety level daily, as well as the situations that trigger these feelings
- Listing positive activities and tracking their completion daily
- Developing an "action plan" for both the caregiver and care-recipient to implement skill practice
- Using a thought record to examine and alter negative thinking patterns about caregiving
- Completing the health passport *Mi Guia de Salud* ("My Health Guide"), in which caregivers record specific details related to their medical check-ups, medications taken, and medical providers' contact information

- Developing a "maintenance plan," which involves asking caregivers to think about situations or events likely to occur in the next few months that will cause stress and recording skills learned in the program that can be used to help deal with the situation

On the second day, care managers, interventionists, and *promotoras* were brought together to learn the CALMA group program (corresponding to REACH I). They received background information and results from the original REACH I group program. During the training the interventionists participated in live demonstrations of each of the four CALMA group sessions.

Description of the Final Modified Interventions Used in San Diego County

We redesigned the CALMA small group program to include four group sessions to be offered by a trained care manager with assistance from a *promotora*. The care managers acted as lead group facilitators responsible for teaching the skills and exercises covered in the session. The *promotora*s assisted the care managers in various ways, such as walking around the classroom to assist individual caregivers with the exercises and materials (especially for caregivers with literacy issues or needing help writing their responses). We also offered three between-session telephone calls. Care managers would check in with caregivers on how things were going as they were implementing suggested changes and practicing their assigned exercises at home. The four CALMA group sessions encompass the key components from REACH I: managing stress with relaxation exercises; increasing pleasurable activities (i.e., behavioral activation); cognitive restructuring; assertiveness training to help manage anger and frustration; and getting the help one needs. We eliminated certain components from the original protocol because other SCRC services readily offered them. The format of the sessions closely followed the original REACH I procedures. For example, each session started with a review of the previous class material and home practice assignments and ended with an introduction of a new relaxation exercise. Additionally, to ensure program fidelity, we required care managers to audio-record the sessions, which a consultant later reviewed and rated, and both care managers and *promotoras* had opportunities to ask questions and receive feedback from weekly supervision meetings.

The CUIDAR home-based program was redesigned to include four individual home sessions offered by a care manager and three telephone calls in between home sessions (a shortened version of the original REACH II protocol). We tailored each session to the individual caregiver's needs by determining which modules included in the Caregiver's Guide were most relevant and important.

The decision as to which content areas would be covered was based on review of baseline assessment information and consultation with Dr. Gallagher-Thompson, who met by teleconference biweekly with the care managers for the first year of program implementation. Following the original REACH II model, each session took place with the individual caregiver in his or her home and lasted up to 2 hours. The telephone calls provided an opportunity for the care managers to check in and give feedback to the caregivers on the specific skills that were being taught.

Care managers could choose among the following modules:

- Learning to build and maintain a strong social network (*Social Support*)
- Managing caregiver stress by learning to use relaxation exercises (*Managing Stress*)
- Increasing caregiver pleasurable activities (*Pleasant Activities*)
- Restructuring negative or unhelpful thoughts to improve one's mood (*Understanding Your Feelings*)
- Maintaining one's physical health by attending to the caregiver's medical appointments and tracking personal health-related information (*Healthy Life*)
- Home safety tips to reduce potential hazards or injury to dementia patient (*Home Safety*)
- Tips on how to better communicate with someone diagnosed with dementia (*Communicating with Your Loved One*)
- Managing difficult dementia-related behaviors, such as wandering, asking the same question repeatedly, and forgetting names and faces (*My Loved One's Behavior*)

We examined the content to make it specific to the region (e.g., challenges involved in border crossing and whether comparable services would be available in Mexico to those in CA) and improve the look and feel of the materials and make them more user friendly. For example, the Caregiver Guide contained culturally appropriate photos and images throughout and had pockets to insert worksheets for each module. Every module is color-coded and includes a brief introduction to its topic to orient the caregiver to the section. Additionally, we gave special attention to the language used in each module for cultural appropriateness and ensured that the literacy level was maintained at the 6th grade level or lower to meet the average reading level of the target Latino group. Lastly, several modules included a cultural *Dicho*, which is a special idiom or quote known in the Latino culture that is often used to make a point or motivate a change in behavior.

We implemented several measures to maintain fidelity to the original REACH interventions. Consultants again carefully reviewed final materials, and the care managers were required to attend training sessions (described earlier) to learn the steps to deliver the interventions correctly. For both programs, care managers were required to audio-record their sessions for fidelity checks. These were done by Veronica Cardenas, who is a bilingual/bicultural Spanish speaking psychologist who worked on the original REACH projects in northern CA with Dr. Gallagher-Thompson. Feedback was provided to the care managers in a timely manner so that the interventions would be delivered as planned.

We further modified the programs following the initial launch. At first, the four sessions in both programs were to be offered every other week (per consultants' recommendations) as a way to extend the length of contact with caregivers and allow more time for materials to be absorbed and applied to caregivers' situations. The SCRC quickly discovered, however, that a significant number of caregivers were not returning or were missing from sessions. As a result, the four sessions were offered in consecutive weeks—a modification that significantly improved participant retention and satisfaction with the program.

Outcomes

The REACHing Out program has been successful and exceeded target expectations for enrollment. The overall program also was successful in other target outcomes related to caregiver psychological well-being, to be described below. The original target of the Rosalynn Carter Institute for Caregiving was to serve 25 Latino caregivers in one year, whereas San Diego County's goal was to serve 200 Latino caregivers annually for the duration of the contract. Since enrollment began in June 2010 through January 2014 (the period for which data are currently available), a total of 647 caregivers enrolled in CALMA and 39 in CUIDAR. In the 2012–2013 fiscal years alone, the SCRC enrolled 231 Latino caregivers into the combined programs. Thus, these programs appear to have been well received in the Latino communities in southern San Diego County. In fact, they have now become "institutionalized" into the standard SCRC program offerings—a significant milestone that was not anticipated at the outset but is perhaps the most important outcome of this body of work.

In terms of impact of the two programs on the psychological well-being of Latino Alzheimer's disease caregivers, we need to view results in the context of translational research—from ivory tower to community—rather than in the context of traditional academic research. This means we

> *"We need to view results in the context of translational research – from ivory tower to community – rather than in the context of traditional academic research."*

have to examine each program's impact separately, keeping in mind that, contrary to traditional research methods, participants were not randomly assigned to conditions. Instead they were assigned to one program versus the other according to their levels of symptom severity at the baseline assessment, which included self-report measures of depression and perceived "burden" or stress due to caregiving. For instance, caregivers who reported high levels of depression (that is, they scored above a standardized cut-off) were generally offered the CUIDAR program so they could get more individualized help. In contrast, those whose caregiving burden was relatively high but whose depression was low were assigned to CALMA, where the small group interaction could help them learn about others in the same situation and how they were handling similar problems. In general, this system worked out well, and there were few "transfers" between programs.

Demographics

All CALMA ($N = 647$) and CUIDAR ($N = 39$) caregivers were Latinos, with a majority identifying as Mexican or Chicano (87.0 % and 89.7 %, respectively). Most in both programs were female (90.5 % and 97.4 %, respectively). CALMA caregivers tended to be older than CUIDAR caregivers; however, the majority from each program was in the age range from 40 to 59 (58.4 % and 43.6 %, respectively), which is consistent with other research with Latino Alzheimer's disease caregivers.

Program Satisfaction

Caregivers were asked to complete several items to assess the perceived benefits of the program they had received. Most either agreed or strongly agreed that because of the program, they felt more comfortable seeking help (CALMA = 98.3 %; CUIDAR = 97.5 %). Also, virtually all reported that they were satisfied with services received (CALMA = 99.7 %; CUIDAR = 100 %).

Psychological Well-Being Outcomes

Caregivers were interviewed at baseline (upon enrollment at SCRC) and again about 6 months after participating in either CALMA or CUIDAR. A comprehensive intake assessment was done by SCRC staff that included several measures to assess psychological well-being. Of those, we will discuss three: (1) Self-rated health (the extent to which overall health was seen as interfering with caregivers' ability to do what they wanted to do in their daily lives); (2) perceived burden or stress related to caregiving, as indexed by the Zarit Burden Interview; and (3) self-reported symptoms of depression, as indexed by the CES-D scale. The latter two are widely used in caregiver research and were used in the original REACH studies.

Perceived Health

To assess caregiver attentiveness towards his or her own health, a standalone question on the assessment tool was added: "How much does your health stand in the way of you doing the things you want to do?" There were four possible responses: "Not at All," "A Little," "Moderately," and "Very Much." This question was administered during an initial assessment prior to the REACH intervention, and again at a reassessment approximately 6 months later, after caregivers had gone through a 4-week intervention.

CALMA
During the initial assessment, 27.0 % of caregivers in this program reported that their health was either "very much" or "moderately" standing in their way of doing the things they wanted to do. At reassessment only 11.6 % reported this.

CUIDAR
At baseline, 50.0 % of caregivers in this program reported that their health was either "very much" or "moderately" standing in their way of doing the things they wanted to do. At reassessment, virtually none reported this.

Zarit Burden Interview

Caregivers were given the brief (12-item) version of the Zarit Burden Interview [22, 23], which measures perceived burden or stress related to being in the caregiving role. They rated each item on a 5-point scale from 0 (never) to 4 (nearly always), with higher scores indicating greater burden, yielding a possible range of 0–44. "High Burden" is defined as greater than or equal to 8, the cut-off score typically used in research studies.

CALMA
Fewer caregivers reported high levels of burden after participating in the CALMA intervention groups. Only 15 % scored above the cut-off at the reassessment, indicating that burden was reduced for the majority of participants. A paired sample t-test was used to assess change over time and significant reduction was found: mean$=8.02$ at baseline vs. 4.22 at reassessment ($t(380)=19.32, p<0.001$).

CUIDAR
Similarly, the number of caregivers reporting high levels of burden after receiving personalized intervention in the CUIDAR program drastically reduced; at reassessment, less than 10 % were still highly burdened. Note, however, the small sample size; caution should be used in interpreting these data. Again, a paired sample t-test was used to assess change over time, and significant reduction was found: mean$=10.39$ at baseline vs. 2.86 at reassessment ($t(27)=11.06, p<0.001$).

Depression

The Center for Epidemiologic Studies Depression Scale (CES-D) [24] is a 20-item self-report screening tool that assesses for current symptoms of depression. The CES-D has a potential range of 0–60, with higher scores indicating more depressive symptoms; those who score 16 or greater are considered to be experiencing a significant level of depression and likely are in need of treatment. This scale has been widely used in prior research with dementia family caregivers, including with Latino caregivers in the REACH studies.

CALMA
The number of caregivers reporting high levels of depression decreased after participating in this program. At baseline, 55.5 % were at high risk for clinical depression based on CES-D score, whereas at the reassessment only 26.6 % were at high risk. The paired sample t test showed significant reduction over time: the mean dropped from 18.18 to 11.88 ($n=452$; t $(451)=13.38$, $p<0.001$).

CUIDAR
A similar reduction in the percentage of caregivers scoring above the clinical cut-off for depression is found here: at baseline, 76.7 % were at high risk, while at the reassessment only 10.0 % were at high risk. This finding must be evaluated in light of the fact that CUIDAR participants were selected partly on the basis of high distress in terms of initial depression level, so it is not surprising that such a high percent were clinically depressed at the outset. What is noteworthy is the highly significant drop in this percentage over time. As well, the overall mean score here dropped from 22.36 to 8.57 ($n=28$; t $(27)=9.55$, $p<0.001$).

Lessons Learned

A key factor to the success of these projects was implementation of the "Confianza Triangle" (see Fig. 9.1) from the beginning. The *promotoras'* active participation in development of materials, training sessions, and many meetings where we talked about how best to implement these programs was critical to the programs' success. The many challenges to engaging Latino caregivers in treatment have been well documented in the literature [21, 25], and we are certain that without the *promotoras'* help with outreach and engagement, the programs would not have been as successful as they turned out to be. At the same time, the use of *promotoras* in outreach (especially when they are not employees of the lead agency) can be a challenge. To address this challenge with the four *promotoras* assigned to the program (who were employed by *La Maestra* Community Health Center and San Ysidro Health Centers), we took multiple steps. For example, formal sub-contract agreements were created and signed by the partner agency executives along with the SCRC's executive team. These agreements detailed the partnership and described the original REACH programs, the role of the *promotoras,* and the expected annual compensation to the partner agencies. We created and reviewed job descriptions and provided special trainings to teach about the original REACH models and what we wanted the new programs to achieve. Due to significant staff turnover in these jobs, this training followed a formal curriculum. Additionally, we held regular, structured meetings to review goals, referrals, outreach activities, and activity logs for reporting purposes and to answer questions and address concerns.

The annual outreach goals ($N=400$ unduplicated clients) for the *promotoras* (described as "prevention activities") and the intervention goals ($N=230$ unduplicated clients) for the care managers up to today are very clear and restricted to the South Bay region of San Diego County. Over the program's 5-year history, the quality of outreach contacts and referrals has improved dramatically. Roughly 9 % of all outreach contacts become referrals to the interventions. Of the referrals, approximately 47 % go through the assessment portion of the program; of those assessed, over 80 % participate and graduate from the program. Due to the restricted target region, *promotoras* tend to be very competitive in their outreach efforts. There is great pride in knowing that he or she made a quality referral and that the individual referred graduated from the program. In addition, the *promotoras* assist the care managers in the CALMA small group program, and they become a familiar face to many of the participants. To encourage healthy competition and minimize conflicts, we created a *promotora* coordinator position (with funding from the county) to better coordinate outreach efforts, provide mentorship and supervision, and mitigate competitive conflicts (e.g., overlapping territories, encroaching on another *promotora's* community contact). This coordinator now meets weekly with the team of *promotoras* to review goals, referrals, outreach activities, activity logs for reporting purposes, answer questions, address concerns, and review a spreadsheet with the team that highlights referrals and graduates per *promotora*. This coordinator, plus SCRC's director of education and programs, also meets with the extended group monthly—consisting of the *promotoras* themselves, their agency supervisors, and SCRC's two care managers. This has really helped to improve communications among all the principal parties and helps keep the programs "on track."

Overall, it is important to point out that through these processes and respectful listening to all stakeholders time and time again, we all learned how to work effectively together. This required flexibility and good communication to ensure that clear lines of communication were established to address problems, issues, and concerns in a timely manner. The SCRC learned that there is an ongoing need for training and supervision of all staff on the project, including management at partner agencies. The SCRC had to recognize and adjust expectations of productivity, because the turnover for *promotoras* was high. Meanwhile, the staff learned how to maximize their time to meet the project goals. Also, our community partners learned that in their work promoting the "new REACH," they could also meet their own goals of obtaining referrals for their agencies.

One Partner's Perspective: Delores Gallagher-Thompson

On a more personal level, all the researchers on the team (including me) learned that we can negotiate differences between the "ivory tower" and the "real world" in ways that respect the very different contexts we are coming from and, at the same time, develop products and services that are faithfully grounded in evidence-based principles and practices. For me, this was a remarkable, impactful learning experience—it was the first time in my professional career that I worked in such a "hands-on" way with so many different community partners who were located so far away. My previous experience focused on smaller agencies and programs in the greater San Francisco Bay area—we had our challenges and issues, of course, but because the teams were smaller and closer together geographically, resolutions were easier to come by. For REACHing Out, a number of in-person trips to the San Diego area were necessary, as well as very frequent teleconference calls and online exchanges. This experience taught me a number of skills that were rooted in its very challenges—for example, how to communicate clearly when I was not there in person and I needed to rely on electronic media to get my points across. Most importantly, it taught me how to listen well to what was being said and really pause and think before expressing opinions or recommendations. I was particularly sensitive to the fact that because I was non-Latino (in my heritage, though very Latina in my cultural preferences!), I had to listen harder and think more before speaking out. These are important lessons that I have since had the privilege to apply in other contexts—for example, training providers in Australia in the use of another derivative caregiver program (also based in the original REACH models) through use of Skype and videoconferencing. This experience would never have been one I would have done without the prior experience with REACHing Out that thoroughly prepared me for that work.

To analyze in advance the SCRC's organization capacity was another important key to the success of these programs. It was imperative to ensure that the SCRC was ready to serve the Latino population and that it had the capacity to offer culturally appropriate services. As mentioned earlier, in order to assess for this capacity, outside experts were employed to evaluate where the organization was at the time. It was also important to keep in mind the cost to implement these programs and if this cost was manageable. In addition, it was crucial to ensure that the program being built was capable of being sustainable. A key step for sustainability was establishing collaborative partnerships with organizations in the community who were already serving the population we were looking to serve. Having discussions with these organizations early on and then creating formal partnerships with them helped tremendously during the planning and implementation phases and, later, with sustainability. Lastly, collecting impact data (using reliable measures that have been often used in caregiving research) has helped enormously to demonstrate to the funding sources, and to other interested parties, that REACHing Out is a successful model that provides tangible results and improves people's lives.

Among the lessons learned for future projects is the need to create and implement proper documentation of the procedures and protocols at the beginning. Also, having an advisory committee that is open and flexible to change that inevitably accompanies the growth of the program proved to be an important collaboration. Maintaining open lines of communication between the researchers on the committee and the organization itself (as well as the community stakeholders) was another key factor. SCRC's management team educated the researchers regarding the San Diego geography and SCRC's capacity in terms of carrying out the project. Meanwhile, the researchers rolled up their sleeves on this project and adjusted their scientific expectations based on the feedback provided by SCRC and other community partners. For the academic partners, much has been learned in the process of implementing the REACH interventions in a real-world community setting. For instance, it was crucial to listen to feedback provided on the feasibility of replicating the exact same treatment models in a new environment with a different set of resources and a different target population. Additionally, academic partners balanced the need to make the programs "feasible" with the equally important need to stay true to the original model and thoughtfully consider what the key features were that had to remain. Following multiple consultations (as described above), once the best intervention models were determined, academic partners worked with SCRC to create a good "fit" between staff and caregivers. For example, staff were bilingual, bicultural, and of the same community where the caregivers resided. Academic partners also created training plans for new staff to learn how to implement the programs, and a fidelity plan to promote high quality protocol adherence.

A final lesson learned is that the burden, stress, and depression associated with dementia family caregiving can be relieved through relatively cost-effective means. Results from CALMA (the small group program) were of clinically meaningful magnitude at much less expense, compared to the home-based CUIDAR program. This underscores the importance of doing a careful caregiver assessment at the outset so that the more expensive and time-consuming services can be reserved for those who truly need them.

Future Directions

As of this writing, most of the partnerships mentioned are still active. Currently the communities being served are in close proximity to the US-Mexico border and Tijuana, Mexico. This southern part of San Diego County includes the city of San Ysidro, which is one of the busiest land border-crossings and where services are most needed. One recommendation from these findings is that funders, in collaboration with SCRC, expand this program to northern San Diego County that also has a substantial Latino population. SCRC plans to continue to lobby San Diego County for additional funding to enable this program expansion to occur. We all need to recognize that dementia is a global problem; its incidence and prevalence are rapidly rising [26]. Future partnerships with other agencies throughout the United States and even with other countries around the world would be invaluable in expanding these services to other communities that have a large Latino population with relatively low health literacy and low socio-economic status who nevertheless have significant (often unmet) service needs.

SCRC is now actively working to create a toolkit based on our new models to disseminate so that other organizations can benefit from our experience and lessons learned. The toolkit will include training materials and protocols to help build other organizations' capacity. This should allow other community-based providers to replicate and benefit from the translational research that we have implemented, and would allow more evidence-based programs to reach populations who need them the most.

Acknowledgment This narrative is based upon work supported and funded by San Diego County Behavioral Health Services and the Rosalynn Carter Institute. The authors would like to thank Marissa Goode from the University of California San Diego for her assistance in statistical data analyses for this narrative.

References

1. World Health Organization, Alzheimer's Disease International. Dementia: A Public Health Priority. 2012; Available from: http://whqlibdoc.who.int/publications/2012/9789241564458_eng.pdf.
2. Administration on Aging. A statistical profile of Hispanic older Americans aged 65+. Department of Health & Human Services; 2010 [cited 2013 March 5]; Available from: http://www.aoa.gov/AoARoot/Aging_Statistics/minority_aging/Facts-on-Hispanic-Elderly.aspx.
3. American Psychiatric Association. Diagnostic and statistical manual of mental disorders fifth edition (DSM-5). 5th ed. Washington, DC: American Psychiatric Association; 2013.
4. Alzheimer's Association. Minorities Contract Alzheimer's Earlier. 2011; Available from: http://www.elderauthority.com/alzheimers-association-en-espanol.
5. Clark CM, DeCarli C, Mungas D, Chui HI, Higdon R, Nuñez J, et al. Earlier onset of Alzheimer disease symptoms in Latino individuals compared with Anglo individuals. Arch Neurol. 2005;62(5):774–8.
6. Hinton L, Chambers D, Velásquez A. Making sense of behavioral disturbances in persons with dementia: Latino family caregiver attributions of neuropsychiatric inventory domains. Alzheimer Dis Assoc Disord. 2009;23(4):401–5.
7. Alzheimer's Association. Alzheimer's Disease Facts and Figures. 2013 [cited 2013 september 2]; Available from: http://www.alz.org/downloads/facts_figures_2013.pdf.
8. Pinquart M, Sörensen S. Ethnic differences in stressors, resources, and psychological outcomes of family caregiving: a meta-analysis. Gerontologist. 2005;45(1):90–106.
9. Vitaliano PP, Zhang J, Scanlan JM. Is caregiving hazardous to one's physical health? A meta-analysis. Psychol Bull. 2003;129(6):946–72.
10. Vitaliano PP, Young HM, Zhang J. Is caregiving a risk factor for illness? Curr Direct Psychol Sci. 2004;13(1):13–6.
11. Savard J, Leduc N, Lebel P, Beland F, Bergman H. Caregiver satisfaction with support services: influence of different types of services. J Aging Health. 2006;18(1):3–27.

12. Alvarez P, Rengifo J, Emrani T, Gallagher-Thompson D. Latino older adults and mental health: a review and commentary. Clin Gerontol. 2014;37(1):33–48.
13. McHenry JC, Insel KC, Einstein GO, Vidrine AN, Koerner KM, Morrow DG. Recruitment of older adults: success may be in the details. The Gerontologist. 2012 Aug 16 (Epub ahead of print).
14. Schulz R, Burgio L, Burns R, Eisdorfer C, Eisdorfer C, Gallagher-Thompson D, Gitlin LN, et al. Resources for enhancing Alzheimer's Caregiver Health (REACH): overview, site-specific outcomes, and future directions. Gerontologist. 2003;43(4):514–20.
15. Gallagher-Thompson D, Coon DW, Solano N, Ambler C, Rabinowitz Y, Thompson LW. Change in indices of distress among Latino and Anglo female caregivers of elderly relatives with dementia: site-specific results from the REACH national collaborative study. Gerontologist. 2003;43(4):580.
16. Belle SH, Burgio L, Burns R, Coon D, Czaja SJ, Gallagher-Thompson D, et al. Enhancing the quality of life of dementia caregivers from different ethnic or racial groups. Ann Intern Med. 2006;145(10):727–38.
17. Mental Health Services Act. Proposition 63. [cited 2014 April 19]; Available from: http://prop63.org/about/prop-63-today/.
18. Valle R, Garrett Mario D, Velasquez R. Developing dementia prevalence rates among Latinos: a locally-attuned, data-based, service planning tool. J Popul Ageing. 2013;6(3):211–25.
19. Haan MN, Mungas DM, Gonzalez HM, Ortiz TA, Acharya A, Jagust WJ. Prevalence of dementia in older Latinos: the influence of type 2 diabetes mellitus, stroke and genetic factors. J Am Geriatr Soc. 2003;51(2):169–77.
20. Mausbach B, Coon D, Depp C, Rabinowitz Y, Wilson-Arias E, Kraemer H, et al. Ethnicity and time to institutionalization of dementia patients: a comparison of Latina and Caucasian female family caregivers. J Am Geriatr Soc. 2004;52(7):1077–84.
21. Gallagher-Thompson D, Singer LS, Depp C, Mausbach BT, Cardenas V, Coon DW. Effective recruitment strategies for Latino and Caucasian dementia family caregivers in intervention research. Am J Geriatr Psychiatry. 2004;12(5):484–90.
22. Zarit SH, Orr NK, Zarit JM. The hidden victims of Alzheimer's disease: families under stress. New York: New York University Press; 1985.
23. Bedard M, Molloy DW, Squire L, Dubois S, Dubois S, Lever JA, O'Donnell M. The Zarit Burden interview: a new short version and screening version. Gerontologist. 2001;41(5):652–7.
24. Radloff LS. The CES-D Scale: a self-report depression scale for research in the general population. Appl Psychol Meas. 1977;1(3):385–401.
25. Gallagher-Thompson D, Solano N, Coon D, Areán P. Recruitment and retention of Latino dementia family caregivers in intervention research: issues to face, lessons to learn. Gerontologist. 2003;43(1):45–51.
26. Gallagher-Thompson D, Tzuang YM, Au A, Brodaty H, Charlesworth G, Gupta R, et al. International perspectives on nonpharmacological best practices for dementia family caregivers: a review. Clin Gerontol. 2012;35(4):316–55.

Narrative 10
Implementing a Peer Support Program for Veterans: Seeking New Models for the Provision of Community-Based Outpatient Services for Posttraumatic Stress Disorder and Substance Use Disorders

Shaili Jain, Kaela Joseph, Hannah Holt, Craig S. Rosen, and Steven E. Lindley

This is the story of physicians and health professionals who came together to establish the Peer Support Program, to develop new models for the provision of community based outpatient services where capacity of the system and providers is challenged to meet a community's needs.

S. Jain, M.D. (✉) • S.E. Lindley, M.D., Ph.D.
VA Palo Alto Health Care System, Menlo Park, CA, USA

Department of Psychiatry and Behavioral Sciences, Stanford University School of Medicine, Stanford, CA, USA
e-mail: sjain1@stanford.edu; lindleys@stanford.edu

K. Joseph, M.S.
VA Palo Alto Health Care System, Menlo Park, CA, USA
e-mail: kaela.joseph@gmail.com

H. Holt, M.S.
Department of Clinical Psychology, Palo Alto University, Palo Alto, CA, USA
e-mail: hholt@paloaltou.edu

C.S. Rosen, Ph.D.
VA Palo Alto Health Care System, Menlo Park, CA, USA

Department of Psychiatry and Behavioral Sciences, Stanford University School of Medicine, Stanford, CA, USA

National Center for PTSD Dissemination and Training Division, Menlo Park, CA, USA
e-mail: craig.rosen@va.gov

© Springer International Publishing Switzerland 2015   125
L.W. Roberts et al. (eds.), *Partnerships for Mental Health*,
DOI 10.1007/978-3-319-18884-3_10

Defining the Issue

More than 3.4 million rural[1] veterans are enrolled in the VA health care system [1]. Men and women from geographically rural and highly rural areas make up a disproportionate share of service members, comprising about one third (32 %) of the enrolled veterans who served in the recent conflicts in Afghanistan and Iraq, referred to here as Operation Enduring Freedom (OEF), Operation Iraqi Freedom (OIF), and Operation New Dawn (OND) veterans. Many of these soldiers are returning to their rural communities [1], and there is a shortage of mental health professionals practicing in rural areas. Hence, rural veterans face significant disparities in accessing care, especially highly specialized services [2].

Rural veterans with depression and anxiety disorders are significantly less likely to receive psychotherapy services, and when they do receive them, the amount provided is limited, relative to rural veterans' urban counterparts [3]. While telehealth and other technological interventions are successful strategies to address some of these issues [4], geographical inequities in the availability and distribution of mental health professionals are unlikely to change in the near future [5].

Effectively treating veterans with posttraumatic stress disorder (PTSD) in a timely manner remains a pressing public health concern. Up to 13 % of OEF/OIF/OND veterans have combat-related PTSD [6, 7]. Despite the availability of evidence-based treatments, which ameliorate core PTSD symptoms and prevent further negative consequences such as substance use disorders (SUDs) and suicide [8, 9], help-seeking veterans often do not follow up with the recommended course of psychological [10] or pharmacological [11] therapies. This may be due, in part, to problems at the interface between the veteran and the health care system. Recent research suggests that veterans with PTSD are less likely to perceive their health care experience as being positive [12] and that negative perceptions of mental health care (e.g., lack of trust in mental health professionals) predicts low service utilization [13].

Further, research has found that veterans' concerns about treatments are larger barriers than stigma, emotional readiness, or logistical issues [14]. These concerns include being misunderstood by clinicians or belief that medications will not relieve their symptoms [14]. For veterans who live in rural communities, studies suggest that the rural culture itself may foster a perceived need for greater self-reliance, independence, and conformity to social norms (whether positive or negative toward mental health treatments) and thereby delay identification of mental health problems and discourage the use of formal mental health services [15, 16]. Finally, OEF/OIF/OND veterans are less likely to present in mental health outpatient treatment than veterans from previous eras [5] and may be prone to prematurely dropping out of PTSD treat-

---

[1] The US Census defines *rural* as "territory, population, and housing units not classified as Urban" and defines *urban* as "comprising all territory, population, and housing units in urbanized areas and in places of 2,500 or more persons outside urbanized areas."

ment altogether [10, 11]. In light of these challenges, there is a pressing need for innovative interventions that focus on enhancing the reach of PTSD treatment, that is, making treatments more accessible and easier to engage in and adhere to [17].

Toward an Approach/Solution

Involving peer support in the care of rural veterans is an innovative solution [18, 19]. Peer support providers have personal experience with mental illness and have attained significant improvements in their own condition. Peer support programs offer formal services and support to a peer considered to be not as far along in his or her own recovery process. Consistent with this definition, and integral to the peer support process, is that the peer support providers reveal their experiences with mental illness and specifically focus on the skills, strengths, supports, and resources they used in their recovery. Peer support is considered a form of health care, with peer support providers acting as members of the mental health care team [19, 20]. While the use of peer support to provide services to individuals living with serious mental illness, such as bipolar disorder and schizophrenia, has been well investigated, the use of such an intervention for individuals with PTSD is a relatively new concept [21, 22]. We have previously postulated that the principal mechanisms of action of such a peer support intervention are (1) the promotion of social bonds, (2) the promotion of recovery, and (3) the promotion of knowledge about the health care system [23].

"We are not suggesting that peers replace the evidence-based psychotherapies and pharmacotherapies for PTSD and SUDs offered by qualified mental health professionals but, rather, that they provide innovative supplemental services that aim to engage those with PTSD and SUDs in treatment long enough that they might experience benefit from professionally delivered treatment. Also, because these peers come from the same rural community as the patients they are serving, this shared background may be helpful in combating some of the stigma associated with the decision to seek mental health services."

With regard to care delivered in rural regions, peers can potentially play a key role in augmenting the PTSD and substance use disorders (SUD) care offered by overburdened mental health professionals. We are not suggesting that peers replace the evidence-based psychotherapies and pharmacotherapies for PTSD and SUDs offered by qualified mental health professionals but, rather, that they provide innovative supplemental services that aim to engage those with PTSD and SUDs in treatment long enough that they might experience benefit from professionally delivered treatment. Also, because these peers come from the same rural community as the patients they are serving, this shared background may be helpful in combating some of the stigma associated with the decision to seek mental health services.

Introducing the Partners

Mr. Guy Holmes, a Peer Support Program employee since March 2012, is a Vietnam veteran from Sonora, CA, who works 20 hours/week providing peer support services at the VA Sonora clinic. Mr. Erik Ontiveros, a Peer Support Program employee since April 2013, is an Iraq war veteran who provides peer support services at the VA clinics in Stockton and Modesto, CA, 20 hours/week. Kaela Joseph and Hannah Holt have provided administrative and research assistance for the program. William Boddie is a licensed clinical social worker responsible for providing clinical supervision for the certified peer specialists. Dr. Shaili Jain and Dr. Steven Lindley are both psychiatrists and provide administrative leadership and direction for the program. In addition to these partners, the program has the following consultants: Craig Rosen, a health services researcher and deputy director of the National Center for PTSD; Darryl Silva, senior mental health administrator for the Stockton, Modesto, and Sonora Community Based Outpatient Clinics and national director of VA Peer Support Services, located in the VA central office.

A private donation from the Michael Alan Rosen Foundation solely funds the certified peer specialist and program support assistant positions. The funding is primarily used to support the salaries, benefits, and associated costs of the peer specialist and the part-time program support assistant. Additional associated costs include peer specialist training and financial support for outreach efforts and mileage. Along with the Michael Alan Rosen Foundation, Stanford and the VA contribute resources towards the program's support, such as the time of Dr. Lindley and Dr. Jain for project leadership and the computers, servers, telephones, administrative support, office supplies, and workspaces already in place at VA clinics.

Getting Started

In early 2012, we developed the Peer Support Program as a clinical demonstration project at the Sonora Community Based Outpatient Clinic of the VA Palo Alto Healthcare System. During the initial stages we relied on the existing support and infrastructure provided by the national VA Peer Support Services to guide many decisions for implementing the procedures and policies related to this project. Program leadership and direction came from the Menlo Park campus of this health care system, which is located 130 miles from Sonora. The Sonora clinic serves more than 3500 veterans in the Sierra Nevada Foothills, a rural region of Northern California, and its services include mental health, general medicine, social work, substance abuse, and wellness. The majority of veterans seeking services at the clinic are male (93 %) and Caucasian (75 %), and their average age is 61 years. The most common primary diagnosis at the Sonora clinic is PTSD (49 %), and 19 % of veterans have a secondary diagnosis of SUD. Prior to implementing the program, the clinic employed a mental health team that included two full-time general mental health social workers and one OEF/OIF case manager. All psychiatry appointments are conducted through telemental health, unless the veteran opts to commute to another VA clinic for psychiatric care. In light of the success of this demonstration project, in April 2013 the program was expanded to the Stockton and Modesto Community Based Outpatient Clinics, both in underserved regions of Northern California that serve patients who reside in rural areas.

"The rural clinics are busy," offers William Boddie, the clinical social worker and supervisor for the certified peer specialists. "It feels like we are putting out fires constantly." The biggest challenges he encounters in his daily work for the Peer Support Program are managing referrals to overbooked mental health professionals and engaging veterans in treatment. He continues, "The peer specialists are in a unique position to help with both of these challenges." Boddie helps the peer specialists communicate with other mental health providers and integrates their peer support services with the rest of the veterans' care, thus supporting and augmenting existing mental health services. Boddie says, "I couldn't do my job without the peer specialists. The role of Erik and Guy [certified peer specialists] is crucial in connecting to veterans who have experienced very painful circumstances. I can relate to my patients as a clinician, but the peer can relate on their level. No matter how much training I have as a licensed clinical social worker, I will never be able to share their experience."

An important first step in implementing the Peer Support Program was to recruit the peers who would provide services. We employed rigorous screening and hiring procedures in accordance with previous recommendations [24, 25]. The clinics' senior mental health administrator was actively involved in the recruitment process and remains an important consultant to the program. Ensuring our peers received adequate training for the position and demonstrated certain competencies was the top priority [18, 19, 26]. Essential components of the peer training were (1) understanding and respecting therapeutic boundaries, (2) active listening, and (3) training in psychological crisis management. We aimed to avoid the use of a rigid didactic training, which may have undermined the natural, unique skills that the peers brought to the treatment team [27, 28].

In addition to running peer support groups, the certified peer specialist provides support via telephone and individual "engagement" visits, if requested by veteran patients. Although the peer conducts his groups independently, a licensed mental health professional is required to be available, on site, at all times, while the peer is interfacing with veteran patients. The peer specialist completes chart reviews and documents all his contacts with the veterans.

The peer is required to engage in weekly supervision with a licensed mental health professional. Supervision typically focuses on one or more of the following domains: components of recovery, professional ethics, customer service, outreach efforts, personal self-development, enhancing communication and group facilitation skills, management of stigma, comprehension of mental illness, recovery tools, professional development, and crisis management. Boddie has had extensive experience supervising students in clinical social work and has much of the same discussions during supervision with the peer specialists as with his other supervisees. Discussion and reflection about ethical considerations and boundaries are important to any mental health provider, but the focus in Boddie's supervision with the peer providers is often how to coach veterans on the basis of the peer specialists' own experience of recovery using available resources and tools. Shaili Jain provides additional supervision through monthly team conference calls and notes that the level of passion and commitment that the peer specialists bring to the team are highly valuable and unique. Dr. Jain admires the peer specialists' commitment to service and their focus on the patient experience. Working in a large health care system with many levels of administrative and regulatory demands can get distracting for clinicians. She reflects, "The peers really want to be of service and are so focused on their patients. It is very refreshing and inspiring."

Another important role for the peer is conducting community outreach, including outreach letters to therapists in the community and personalized letters/flyers to veterans to enhance awareness of the Peer Support Program. Outreach also includes personal appearances at local colleges, job fairs, community events that honor local veterans, and connecting with rural outreach counselors and counselors at the larger hospital system to promote awareness of the program. "The outreach came about organically," states Dr. Jain. "The peer support providers both felt it was an important part of their job and an aspect that most busy mental health professional just do not have time for." One of the advantages of the peer specialists is that they are not burdened by organizational requirements (e.g., billing and charting paperwork) so that they have more time to provide this valuable adjunctive service.

In June 2013, the peer specialists began conducting a focused telephone outreach to Iraq/Afghanistan veterans from the central valley and Sonora area who were not currently engaged in mental health services but had been diagnosed with PTSD and SUD. During these telephone calls, the specialist described the peer support program to his veteran peers and invited them to attend. The specialists both wrote personal letters describing their own journey of recovery and mailed invitations to the peer support program, along with peer support brochures, to this target population.

Erik Ontiveros, one of the certified peer specialists, has cited that dispelling stigma and mistrust is the signature challenge of his work in peer support. As a veteran himself, he recognizes that the culture of the military does not generally lend support to the admission of having a problem or asking for help. Ontiveros overcomes this challenge by using his own experience of difficulty asking for help as an example for the veterans and normalizing their feelings of hesitance about seeking help. He reported that whenever a new group member is present in his support group, he takes the time to share the story of his own treatment and successful recovery after returning home from service. Ontiveros asks the other group members to share their backgrounds and perspectives about how the group has been helpful. He wants the veterans to know that they are not alone and that their hesitation about seeking treatment or help is natural.

Even when veterans have not yet attended one of his peer support groups, Ontiveros still tries to engage veterans over the phone, leaving voicemails and reminding them that help is available when they are ready. Because Ontiveros has been through the process himself, at one point reluctant to accept help after returning home from deployment, he has more empathy for the veterans, which quells any frustration. He also offers that sometimes he will see a veteran in one of his groups who will tell him, "I got your messages and I'm ready now." Ontiveros has to remind himself that even if he never speaks with a veteran directly while conducting telephone outreach, it does not mean that the veteran is not getting the messages or that they are not having an effect.

Program Outcomes

The program keeps detailed records of the peer specialists' clinical activities. The peer specialists and their clinical supervisor complete tracking sheets, and the program assistant compiles data from these forms into various databases to keep track of program outcomes. Veterans who participate in the program are also asked periodically to fill out satisfaction surveys, which are logged into a database and analyzed for quality assurance. In addition to ongoing direct clinical supervision, the entire Peer Support Program team (which is geographically dispersed) meets monthly via conference calls and annually via an in-person retreat.

As of April 30, 2014, the program served 185 veterans (127 in Sonora and 58 in Modesto and/or Stockton), and the peer specialists provided a total of 258 peer support groups, with an average of 10 patients in each group. The 2013 telephone outreach effort identified 148 veterans who were not engaged in mental health treatment. Of those veterans, 87 were successfully contacted by phone, 58 were sent information in the mail, and 3 were contacted by other means. Forty-seven veterans agreed to engage in the Peer Support Program, and an additional 21 indicated they might be interested. The peer specialists have spent almost 300 hours engaging in telephone outreach.

In addition to these services, the peer specialists have provided 188 individual "engagement" visits and conducted more than 200 hours of active community outreach. Clinical supervision for the peer specialists is conducted weekly and usually lasts 1 hour. Holmes, the original peer support specialist, has documented 53 supervision sessions, and Ontiveros, who joined the team later, has documented 27 supervision sessions.

Preliminary patient feedback shows that 75 % of veterans rated the peer services they received as "always" helpful. Also, 75 % of veterans reported that the peer specialist "frequently" provides high quality emotional support, with 25 % reporting the support as "always" being of high quality. Early ratings of peer support group cohesion are encouraging, with veteran patients consistently highly rating the group cohesion and value of the peer support groups. Below are some comments transcribed from anonymous patient feedback of the group experience:

> "*I feel this group meeting is highly beneficial to me.*"
> "*He* [the certified peer specialist] *respects our statements and leads us in a constructive way.*"
> "*I wish I didn't have to wait for over 40 years to be in a group like this.*"

Several striking stories of success and recovery have come from the Peer Support Program. Ontiveros described a female veteran who made a dramatic transformation over a year of attending peer support groups. The veteran used to sit and listen very attentively to the other veterans but never offered her own perspective or shared her experience with PTSD and other mental health problems. Whereas she was very uncomfortable when she first starting to attend the peer support groups, Ontiveros states that she now often shares her feelings and offers advice to other veterans about coping skills. He has noticed a dramatic shift in her level of confidence, especially as she is often the only female in a group of service members who are mostly men. Ontiveros noted that she has been able to recognize that her pain and her experiences of the military are just as valid as those of the male veterans.

Dr. Jain recalled an experience several months into the implementation of the peer support program that gave her a perspective on the power of the program. During a team call, one of the peer specialists mentioned that a veteran who had been determined to be at high risk for suicide had not been to the clinic to see his provider or attended the peer support group for quite some time. The peer specialist added that he had been meeting with this veteran at the local coffee shop. Dr. Jain reported that as the project director, her "red flags were going off," and she became concerned about potential boundary violations and the serious implications of services taking place outside of the clinic. The peer specialist subsequently explained, however, that there is only one coffee shop in this rural town and that he happened to see the veteran there each week when he got his morning coffee. He had not been engaging with the veteran per se, but he could at least offer the veteran a quick "hello" and report back that the veteran was doing well. Dr. Jain realized that overlapping roles would be inevitable in such a rural community. The informal feedback that the peer specialist was able to provide (e.g., that the veteran was fine) was a desirable consequence of him belonging to the same community as the veterans whom he served. The professional boundaries of which Dr. Jain had been trained to be mindful did not entirely map on to the roles that the peer specialists have with veteran patients. The flexibility in the role is part of the unique value that the peers bring to the treatment team.

The Peer Support Program is innovative because, to the best of our knowledge, it is the first program in the US that utilizes peer support specifically to address the needs of individuals living with PTSD. The program is also unique in its deployment of a telephone outreach intervention targeted toward a particular subset of the population identified by the VA databases as being disengaged in treatment. The program also seeks to combine research and practice, keeping detailed records of supervision of the peer specialists' clinical activities and patient satisfaction surveys.

Lessons Learned

Initially, a low number of OIF/OEF/OND veterans used the Peer Support Program. We noted a significant increase in the percentage of visits by these veterans approximately 10 months after the program started. This increase was likely due to time the peer specialists spent conducting engagement visits with veterans who were initially ambivalent about attending peer support groups. These individual engagement sessions possibly helped ease sources of the veterans' ambivalence and allowed for their subsequent engagement in mental health services on a longer-term basis. Levels of involvement by OIF/OEF/OND veterans have continued to increase and are likely a result of the peer specialists' targeted outreach efforts and word-of-mouth by veterans who utilize the program. It is important to note that these engagement visits are an example of a service that overburdened mental health providers may not be in a position to provide routinely as they work in rural or other regions vulnerable to becoming understaffed with mental health professionals.

We have learned about the vital importance of frequent, clear communication between team members who are not only geographically dispersed but also have different backgrounds, professional disciplines, and approaches to patients. The team members are in regular contact, on a day-to-day basis, via e-mail, voicemail, and instant messages and through electronic medical records. In addition, we have weekly clinical supervision meetings, monthly team conference calls, and an annual team retreat. We feel this attention to communication and the emphasis on a culture of open and transparent dialogue provide a safeguard against adverse events occurring in the team (e.g., team member attrition or miscommunication) and, most importantly, promote the provision of high quality services to patients.

One of the ongoing challenges for Dr. Jain is educating professional providers about the roles of the certified peer specialists and making it clear that they provide psychoeducation and support but not psychiatric or psychological treatment. Sometimes other providers do not fully understand the role of the peer specialists and assume the peers can take on responsibilities that are actually outside of their scope of practice. Within that vein, Dr. Jain also views it as her duty to protect the peer specialists from burnout and to support their ongoing recovery. She encourages self-care, self-monitoring, and pacing, making it clear that the peer providers' well-being is a team priority.

Implementing a new and innovative program also has organizational challenges. Ontiveros noted some initial resistance from the other mental health care providers and often felt like "the third wheel" in the beginning stages of implementation. As veterans began attending the peer support groups and relaying positive feedback to their other mental health care providers, however, he felt that he began to be taken more seriously. He had to show that the model worked by demonstrating success before the other mental health care providers could validate his role and responsibilities.

Finally, the licensed mental health professionals on the team have learned to encompass ideas or treatment approaches from the peer specialists on the team, which may be quite different to other clinical preferences or rationales. Over the 2 years this program has been operational, the health professionals have come to view the input from their peer specialist colleagues as unique and a reflection of the true value they bring to the treatment team. Valuing this diversity within the team is a key ingredient of the success of the program and has contributed immeasurably to it flourishing despite the considerable challenges of the geographical areas and the populations that the program serves.

Future Directions

Our primary emphasis is on expanding clinical services with an aim to have, at minimum, nine peer support groups running on a weekly basis with an average of 10–12 regular participants. The peer specialists play an invaluable role in engaging veterans, who may by ambivalent to seek care in mental health services. We envision that the Peer Support Program will prove to be an innovative modality, via which Iraq and Afghanistan veterans will be able to engage in mental health services. We hope that data from a formalized program evaluation effort will further serve to promote the Peer Support Program as a model for use in other VA and community settings.

Acknowledgements The Peer Support Program is funded by a donation from the Michael Alan Rosen Foundation. The authors would also like to acknowledge the efforts of the Peer Support Program clinical team: Certified Peer Specialists Guy Holmes, Erik Ontiveros, and William Boddie, LCSW.

References

1. U.S. Department of Veterans Affairs, Veterans Health Administration Office of Rural Health. Fact Sheet, Information about the Office of Rural Health and Rural Veterans [Internet]. Washington (DC). 2001 Nov-[cited 2014 May 29]. Available from: http://www.ruralhealth.va.gov. Last accessed 15 July 2001
2. Johnson ME, Brems C, Warner TD, Roberts LW. Rural–urban health care provider disparities in Alaska and New Mexico. Adm Policy Ment Health. 2006;33:504–7.
3. Cully JA, Jameson JP, Phillips LL, Kunik ME, Fortney JC. Use of psychotherapy by rural and urban Veterans. J Rural Health. 2010;26(3):225–33. doi:10.1111/j.1748-0361.2010.00294.x.
4. Grubaugh AL, Cain GD, Elhai JD, Patrick SL, Frueh CB. Attitudes toward medical and mental health care delivered via telehealth applications among rural and urban primary care patients. J Nerv Ment Dis. 2008;196:166–70.
5. Brooks E, Novins DK, Thomas D, Jiang L, Nagamoto HT, Dailey N, et al. Personal characteristics affecting veterans' use of services for posttraumatic stress disorder. Psychiatr Serv. 2002;63(9):862–7.
6. Friedman MJ, Keane TM, Resick PA. In: Friedman MJ, Keane TM, Resick PA, editors. PTSD: Twenty-five years of progress and challenges. New York, NY: The Guilford Press; 2010.
7. Thomas JL, Wilk JE, Riviere LA, McGurk D, Castro CA, Hoge CW. Prevalence of mental health problems and functional impairment among active component and National Guard soldiers 3 and 12 months following combat in Iraq. Arch Gen Psychiatry. 2010;67(6):614–23.
8. McDevitt-Murhy ME, Williams JL, Bracken KL, Fields JA, Monahan CJ, Murphy JG. PTSD symptoms, hazardous drinking, and health functioning among U.S. OEF/OIF veterans presenting to primary care. J Trauma Stress. 2010;23(1):108–11.
9. Pietrzak RH, Goldstein MB, Malley JC, Rivers AJ, Johnson DC, Southwick SM. Risk and protective factors associated with suicidal ideation in Veterans of Operations Enduring Freedom and Iraqi Freedom. J Affect Disord. 2010;123(1–3):102–7.
10. Seal KH, Maguen S, Cohen B, Gima KS, Metzler TJ, Ren L, et al. VA mental health services utilization in Iraq and Afghanistan Veterans in the first year of receiving new mental health diagnoses. J Trauma Stress. 2010;23(1):5–156.
11. Jain S, Greenbaum MA, Rosen CS. Do Veterans with posttraumatic stress disorder receive first-line pharmacotherapy? Results from the longitudinal veterans health survey. Prim Care Companion CNS Disord. 2012;14(2). doi:10.4088/PCC.11m01162.

12. Burnett-Zeigler I, Zivin K, Ilgen MA, Islam K, Bohnert AS. Perceptions of quality of health care among veterans with psychiatric disorders. Psychiatr Serv. 2001;62(9):1054–9.
13. Kim PY, Britt TW, Klocko RP, Riviere LA, Adler AB. Stigma, negative attitudes about treatment, and utilization of mental health care among soldiers. Mil Psychol. 2001;23(1):65–81.
14. Stecker T, Shiner B, Watts BV, Jones M, Conner KR. Treatment-seeking barriers for veterans of the Iraq and Afghanistan conflicts who screen positive for PTSD. Psychiatr Serv. 2013;64(3): 280–3.
15. Fox J, Merwin E, Blank M. De facto mental health services in the rural south. J Health Care Poor Underserved. 1995;6(4):434–68.
16. Weiss L, Dyer AR. Concise guide to ethics in mental health care. Arlington, VA: American Psychiatric Publishing; 2004. p. 167–84.
17. Hoge CW. Interventions for war-related post traumatic stress disorder: meeting veterans where they are. JAMA. 2011;306(5):549–51.
18. Ashcraft L, Anthony WA, Martin C. Training veterans in recovery. Two female veterans share how peer employment training is making a difference in their recovery from PTSD. Behav Healthc. 2007;27(7):12–3.
19. Richardson D, Darte K, Grenier S, Darte K, English A, Sharpe J. The Operational Stress Injury Social Support Program: a peer support program in collaboration between the Canadian Forces and Veterans Affairs Canada. In: Figley CR, Nash WP, editors. Combat stress injury: theory, research, and management. New York, NY: Routledge; 2007.
20. Davidson L, Chinman M, Sells D, Rowe M. Peer support among adults with serious mental illness: a report from the field. Schizophr Bull. 2006;32(3):443–50.
21. Harchik AE, Sherman JA, Hopkins MC, Strouse MC, Sheldon JB. Use of behavioral techniques by paraprofessional staff: a review and proposal. Behav Interv. 1989;4(4):331–57.
22. Brekelbaum T. The use of paraprofessionals in rural development. Community Dev J. 1984;19:232–51.
23. Jain S, McLean C, Adler EP, Lindley SE, Ruzek JI, Rosen CS. Does the integration of peers into the treatment of adults with posttraumatic stress disorder improve access to mental health care? A literature review and conceptual model. J Trauma Stress Disor Treat. 2013;2:3.
24. American Psychiatric Association. Diagnostic and statistical manual of mental disorders. Revised 4th ed. Washington, DC: APA; 2000.
25. Creamer MC, Varker T, Bisson J, Darte K, Greenberg N, Lau W, et al. Guidelines for peer support in high-risk organizations: an international consensus study using the Delphi method. J Trauma Stress. 2012;25:134–41.
26. Chinman M, Lucksted A, Gresen R, Davis M, Losonczy M, Sussner B, et al. Early experiences of employing consumer providers in the VA. Psychiatr Serv. 2008;59(11):1315–21.
27. Neuner F, Onyut PL, Ertl V, Odenwald M, Schauer E, Elbert T. Treatment of posttraumatic stress disorder by trained lay counselors in an African refugee settlement: a randomized controlled trial. J Consult Clin Psychol. 2008;76(4):686–94.
28. Giblin PT. Effective utilization and evaluation of indigenous health care workers. Public Health Rep. 1989;104(4):361–8.

Narrative 11

A Journey of Mutual Growth: Mental Health Awareness in the Muslim Community

Rania Awaad

This is the story of cultural challenges and professional obstacles faced by an early-career physician as a Muslim woman in the psychiatric field.

"Why not, Mom?" I asked. I knew the answer but wanted to hear it from her directly. "Well, it's just that you would make a fantastic surgeon," she responded. "No, really, Mom, what's wrong with psychiatry?" I pushed. She just shrugged. Every now and then, though, I would catch my mother whispering to my father, "What will people say about her?" But when I would ask what was bothering them, they would both deny anything was wrong. Despite their hesitations, my parents were supportive when I decided to pursue psychiatry. Their whispering also eventually stopped when I reminded them how people in our community had plenty to say about me after I traveled abroad alone (unbecoming of "a good Muslim girl") as a young 14-year-old to study Islamic Law. Later, however, my "bravery" was celebrated and I was hailed as a "role model" for all Muslim girls. I reassured my parents I would be fine, even if I was destined to be the only Muslim woman in the psychiatric field.

I really couldn't blame my parents or my community. I, too, was once strongly opposed to the fields of psychology and psychiatry. In fact, I equated them with being nearly heretical. These fields were viewed as notorious for taking God out of

R. Awaad, M.D. (✉)
Department of Psychiatry and Behavioral Sciences, Stanford University School of Medicine, Stanford, CA, USA
e-mail: rawaad@stanford.edu

© Springer International Publishing Switzerland 2015
L.W. Roberts et al. (eds.), *Partnerships for Mental Health*,
DOI 10.1007/978-3-319-18884-3_11

the picture when attempting to explain mental illness. It was upon this belief that I attended my first course on psychiatry in medical school. When I think back to this introductory course, I can still remember rolling my eyes at the instructor—a tall, fashionable blonde woman who always wore short skirts with knee-length boots. I had a hard time connecting with her and could not imagine myself in her place one day. But the content of the course itself, however, was surprisingly interesting and relevant. It was in these early days of medical school that I started realizing psychiatry might actually be the field I was looking for when I went into medicine.

I remember being caught off guard by these recurring thoughts, considering that just months earlier I was a person who refused to take psychology courses as an undergraduate college student because it was a "backwards science that good Muslim girls don't study." So why now was I feeling that the content of this course might be the answer to my search?

Although I did not realize it immediately, this early struggle proved to be crucial for my transformation. I decided to give the field of psychiatry a second chance. Perhaps it was the realization that I had chosen medicine to find additional answers to better solve the community problems I was unable to fully resolve as a well-respected religious teacher and activist. I was starting to appreciate that my previous counseling work was missing a holistic understanding of how to bring healing to people with complex issues, particularly those with mental health problems. One day I had the powerful realization that no amount of legal training or familiarity with the rules of Islam would adequately aid me in helping members of my community if their underlying mental health problems were not first addressed. I began to wonder if there were others in the field who, like myself, had roots in faith-based communities and had attempted to use their psychiatric knowledge to bring healing to those communities.

At the behest of my husband, I decided to take the leap and apply for psychiatry residencies. An influential religious leader in our community, he too had seen his fair share of unaddressed mental illness and urged me to consider becoming a psychiatrist in order to bridge the gap between the world of professional mental health care and our faith community. Not quite ready to share the news of this unconventional track with others, I initially kept my decision private. But as I entered my final year of medical school, everyone close to me was wondering what field I would choose. I prepared myself for an onslaught of disapproval and rolling of eyes as I began announcing to family and friends that I was going to apply to psychiatry residencies. Every time I opened my mouth to answer their inquires, I would quite literally brace myself for criticism.

While I did get some snorts covered up by fake coughs in response to my answer, these were fewer than I expected. Interestingly, most of the responses were along the lines of "Oh, our community needs psychiatrists!" or "I need one of those!" Despite this, I wasn't too sure if my family and friends were just trying to be nice; would they ever really go see a psychiatrist if they needed one? What if I spent the next 4–6 years of training in vain, ultimately serving the mental health needs of every group other than the very one I had originally set out to help?

I decided there was only one way to know for sure. I applied for a small research grant for medical students funded by the National Institute of Mental Health (NIMH) to develop a survey about attitudes and perceptions of mental illness among Muslim women living in the United States. I figured since Muslim women were the very group I hoped to work with in the future, I might as well find out if I had any hope of having them as patients. To my pleasant surprise, my proposal was funded! Taking this step would prove to be the first of many in forming successful academic-community partnerships. Having the academic support to study my own community was incredibly helpful. Without an academic platform from which to conduct research, I would not have been able to truly understand the very community I hoped to one day serve.

My survey received ethics approval from the institutional review board and was posted on the Stanford University School of Medicine website with a cover letter highlighting that I was a female medical student hoping to find out more about how my fellow Muslim sisters felt about mental health care and its practitioners. I then asked friends and managers of online groups that specifically supported Muslim women to forward the survey link to their constituents. My cover letter stated my hopes to have 200–300 Muslim women complete my survey. Considering the results of the handful of studies I could find about Muslims and mental health, however, I knew that no study had topped 50 respondents despite the researchers' best efforts. I had first written 100 respondents as my target goal and then at the last minute switched it to 200–300. Why not dream big, right?

The next morning I opened up my inbox and nearly jumped out of my seat. Every time a survey was completed, a message would be delivered there. According to my inbox, there were 200 responses to my survey! Considering that this survey took place before the heyday of social media (Facebook and the like), I was certain a replicating virus had infected my inbox. As I fought conflicting urges of panic and excitement, I clicked on every single response. They were real! They were from different women from all over the country. In a state of excitement I called my parents, husband, and mentors, who all shared in my confused excitement. I spent the next few weeks going about my work but with my inbox open during every waking moment as I watched in amazement the steady flow of new responses trickling in. A few months later, I closed the survey at a staggering 1299 responses by Muslim women living in the United States.

There was much speculation as to how I had broken every record known about research with the Muslim community in the United States. Perhaps the most telling were the hundreds of unsolicited messages sent to the email address included in my cover letter. Message after message revealed the same thing: relief that this topic was being brought to the forefront and by a Muslim woman "with a recognizable and trusted name." In my eyes, this was the "sign" that I must pursue psychiatry and with excellence and precision. It was also perhaps at this point that my family and friends realized that I might be on the verge of something important. I saw them tuck away their trepidation about me entering a field that "Muslims don't need" and start making encouraging comments that "maybe" I was on to something beneficial to Muslims residing in the United States.

I wish I could say my journey was smooth sailing from that point onwards. This was hardly the case, however. I found that, generally speaking, Muslims consider mental illness a taboo topic to discuss. I would often hear, "Oh, those things don't happen in our community" or "Those things only happen to those who lose faith in God." My nationwide survey confirmed these results, with the majority of women (60–70 %) stating they believed mental illnesses were either the result of the evil eye ('*ayn*), evil spirits (*jinn*), or fate (*qadar*). An overwhelming majority (over 80 %) believed that the cure for mental illnesses was Qur'anic recitation. When asked whom they would go to first, second, and third if they believed they were suffering from a mental illness, mental health providers were either not chosen at all or were chosen last.

> "*Message after message revealed the same thing: relief that this topic was being brought to the forefront and by a Muslim woman 'with a recognizable and trusted name.' In my eyes, this was the 'sign' that I must pursue psychiatry and with excellence and precision. It was also perhaps at this point that my family and friends realized that I might be on the verge of something important. I saw them tuck away their trepidation about me entering a field that 'Muslims don't need' and start making encouraging comments that 'maybe' I was onto something beneficial to Muslims residing in the United States.*"

I just couldn't reconcile the strangeness of these answers with the high levels of educational background of the women who provided them. In fact, most of the women (1000 out of 1299) who took my survey held a Bachelor's degree or higher. I decided to look up statistics about US Muslim women to see if perhaps the online nature of my survey had targeted a particular subgroup of educated Muslim women who were not representative of the majority of Muslim women residing in the United States. I found that according to a landmark study conducted by the Gallup Poll, American Muslim women were one of the most highly educated female religious groups in the United States, second only to American Jewish women. Furthermore, one in three American Muslim women held a professional job, which is equal to the rate of American Muslim men. Thus, as a group, American Muslims had the highest degree of economic gender parity at the high and low ends of the income spectrum. American Muslim women were also equally as likely as men to say they attend the mosque at least once a week. The study concluded that American Muslim women tended to have considerable social influence in their families and communities.

The results of the Gallup Poll study rang true to my experience of the various American Muslim communities in which I had either resided or worked. But how could such educated and influential women hold such strong notions that only faith could treat mental illness? The answer seemed to lie in the disconnect between East and West. The field of psychiatry was seen as a modern, Western construct and "could not possibly help" those following Eastern philosophies. Despite this East–West tension that Muslims were often quick to point out, the candor of the women who wrote the unsolicited messages in response to my anonymous survey (and thus stripped away their veil of anonymity) continued to jab at me. They reminded me that there must be Muslims out there who felt it was time to put tensions and pride aside and take an objective look at some of the issues plaguing the Muslim community.

I owe my renewed dedication to working with the Muslim community to the women who participated in my study. I was truly inspired by their courage and willingness to take the risk and answer questions about such a taboo topic. The study left me with more questions than answers and led to an insatiable urge to pick up the pace of my research and try to find successful ways of connecting more directly with the Muslim community about mental health. I met with my academic mentors as well as my community mentors to discuss more advanced research studies. Here again, the academic-community partnerships I was starting to form proved to be key in providing me with the right balance of mentorship to successfully traverse mostly unchartered territory. It was only through this dual-pronged mentorship that I was truly able to understand how to work with members of the Muslim community who might, in fact, need mental health support but were either in denial of this need or were facing tremendous roadblocks from loved ones around them to accessing care, due to ignorance or fear.

In my third year of psychiatric residency training I was awarded an American Psychiatric Association Minority Fellowship Award. In addition to the outstanding mentorship and networking opportunities it provided, a significant monetary grant also accompanied this fellowship. I chose to use these funds to hire a research assistant who was familiar with classical and modern medical terminology in both the Arabic and English languages to help me access the works of early Muslim scholars about mental illness. All my life I had read and heard, like most other Muslims, that the Golden Era of Islam heralded amazing advancements in all the fields of science and the humanities. From as early as I could remember, I was taught to be proud of my Muslim heritage and its contributions to science, especially medicine. I began to wonder what these great medical works from our past had to say about mental illness. If our noble predecessors were so famous for their forward thinking, solutions, and inventions, perhaps they had once stood at the same crossroads of faith and mental illness as I was standing at now.

By the conclusion of the first year of my fellowship, my research assistant and I had summarized over 115 medical manuscripts, books, and treatises from the seventh to ninth centuries, Islam's Age of Enlightenment. As we sifted through the works of the ancients, we were astounded at how novel the works were for their time. We were amazed to find classifications of mental illnesses that were surprisingly similar to the modern diagnostic manuals of psychiatry. We found sophisticated discussions on the treatment of an array of mental illnesses that most books on the history of mental illness had led us to believe had not appeared until the post-Freudian era. We were struck by the gamut of talk therapies, art therapies, and music therapies and the emphasis on psychiatric milieu that even modern textbooks of psychiatry would have trouble keeping up with. My research assistant and I looked at each other in amazement with each new therapeutic understanding, which was happening almost daily.

These findings prompted us to check out book after book on the history of psychiatry, psychology, and mental illness in an attempt to see if others had made these same discoveries. Every historical account we found, however, either jumped from the Greek and Roman civilization to the twelfth century, completely skipping over the Islamic Golden Era, or only provided a brief or cursory mention of this time period.

Avicenna's *Cannon of Medicine* was perhaps the only book that was consistently mentioned in these historical anthologies because of its fame for having been the primary medical textbook taught in the medical schools of Europe until the sixteenth century. Curiously absent was mention of almost all of the great findings we were discovering. It seemed the progressive work of Muslim physicians from this era remained buried in the dust of time. What little of this knowledge that was translated into English was copied over and over from one book to another, spelling mistakes and all. Eventually, our excitement from finding new proofs of the advancement of the mental health field during the Islamic Golden Era was replaced with the dreadful realization that somehow these important advancements had not reached modern-day Muslims, just as they did not reach historians on the subject. We then understood that Muslims worldwide were not realizing the splendor of their own heritage in this critical medical arena.

Throughout medical school and residency, I received invitations to speak at local and national Islamic conferences and symposia on issues related to Muslim women, female scholarship, Islamic Law, or any combination of the three. These invitations seemed to be accelerated by my appointment as an Adjunct Professor of Islamic Law at the Zaytuna College in Berkeley, CA, during my third year of psychiatry residency. Zaytuna College is the first accredited Muslim liberal arts college in the United States and in its short existence had earned an immense amount of national and international respect and fame among Muslims. I decided to use these speaking engagements with Muslim women as initial opportunities to share facts I was gathering on the history of mental illness in the Muslim world and gauge the response. As I wove the latest find from my research into these talks to hundreds of Muslim women, I noticed the looks of curiosity coupled with sustained attentiveness as I shared my amazement in discovering, for example, that the first psychiatric ward in the entire world was established in ninth century Baghdad as part of the Islamic Hospital System, later becoming a mainstay in Muslim hospitals from that point onwards.

The interest I found among the Muslim women attending these early lectures encouraged me to go forward. I owe my ability to bring a voice to the once silent issue of mental illness wholly to the openness among community members to entertain these discussions. During my lectures I would share how the creation of psychiatric wards in the Muslim world then inspired the creation of standalone psychiatric institutions that became famous for their humane and "moral" treatment of patients, their emphasis on inclusion and not isolation, the introduction of the psychiatric milieu (clean clothes, daily bathing, purposeful activities, healthy diet, and daily visits by physicians) for the mentally ill. These institutions were often in the heart of town, decorated with lavish gardens and flowing fountains (to bring a sense of calm to the ill) and—the real kicker—were fully funded by the Islamic government, which meant that anyone residing in the Muslim lands who was feeling mental turbulence could be treated at these institutions free of charge. The funding came from *zakat* funds, the obligatory yearly alms charity amounting to 2.5 % of a Muslim's saved wealth. Especially to this last point I saw smiles and nods of approval from the audience. I also read surprise on some faces. Most importantly, however, no one stormed out of the room. "I just love talking about our amazing heritage! The synchronizing of the secular and the Divine... the dealing with difficult issues and not hiding from them." From there I would continue on with my original lecture, but with the knowledge that a seed had been planted.

As time went on, Muslim women came up to me after these talks and said they were dealing with anxiety or depression or phobias of one sort or another and didn't know who to talk to for support. They always asked the same question: "Is it true that our faith permits us to see a psychiatrist or psychologist?" They would admit that family and friends had advised them to either talk to the religious leader, Imam, or to just ignore these issues because they would go away on their own eventually. I heard many accounts of *dhikr* (litanies) or dedicated portions of Qur'an these ladies were told to read in hopes of curing their symptoms. When asked if they helped, most answered that they found partial relief in them but wondered if there was more that could be done. Most admitted that they had never had anyone advise them to go to a psychiatrist or psychologist. In fact, if they did hear of psychiatrists and psychologists, it was usually to warn away from them "because they don't understand our ways." Almost every woman I spoke to denied knowing any Muslim mental health professionals.

I learned so much from my conversations with these women. Their courage to bring up very private struggles and difficult questions was incredibly instrumental in opening the door for me to truly understand what my community members were dealing with. Often I was thanked for being a "great teacher," but I would reply in return that it was I who was actually the real student. I consider myself very fortunate to be a pupil of the community.

I also learned from my discussion with members of my community who inquired about mental illness that they experienced a real sense of relief when they learned that not only was it religiously permissible to see a psychiatrist or psychologist (even if he or she were non-Muslim) but that it was the trademark of our Islamic heritage to tear down the barriers between "secular" and "religious." Mental illnesses were paid heed and directly addressed within traditional Muslim societies because of the Qur'anic injunction, "Do not give the property with which God has entrusted you with to the insane, but feed them and clothe them and speak kindly to them" (Qur'an 4:5). There was an understanding that Muslim leaders carried a divine responsibility to ensure proper care for the mentally ill.

Furthermore, the oft-quoted saying of the Prophet Muhammad, peace be upon him, "There is no disease that Allah has created except that He has also created its remedy" was known to be the impetus that caused our noble predecessors to seek out cures, to the best of their ability, for any ailments they encountered. It was clear from our historical records that mental illnesses were not shunned, nor were they belittled. The great Muslim physicians Ar-Razi, Ibn Sina, Al-Balkhi, and countless others had recipe books full of herbal concoctions, various talk therapies, music therapies, and religious invocations for those afflicted by the array of mental illnesses they documented. Woman after woman listened in wonder as I shared this information. Then I would gently suggest she go see a mental health professional in addition to the Imam.

The women I met would usually ask if they could come see me. At that point in time, I was still in training and could not yet take on patients of my own. I promised that as soon as I completed my training, I would dedicate my practice to serving the Muslim community to the best of my ability. I would generally get that hesitant smile back—the one that seemed to say, "Okay, but I won't believe you until it's real."

After graduating from residency and fellowship, I had the opportunity to join the Department of Psychiatry and Behavioral Sciences at Stanford University School of Medicine, where I had trained. My request was twofold: to continue my lines of research, which were just starting to show signs of fruition, and to focus my clinical work to meet the psychiatric needs of the Muslim community residing in the San Francisco Bay Area. After 5 years of training at Stanford and seeing less than a handful of Muslim patients in its outpatient clinics (despite the fact that the Bay Area is home to one of the largest populations of Muslims in the United States), I was certain Muslims were not going to go to a large academic center like Stanford on their own volition for their mental health needs. I realized I needed to go to the Muslim community if I was going to have any amount of success in meeting their mental health needs.

The department chairman, invested in seeing the department form academic-community partnerships, gave the green light for me to search for such community-based clinical opportunities. The timing couldn't have been better. My search coincided with the opening of a new community-based counseling clinic in a neighboring town that was committed to serving the mental health needs of faith-based communities. The founders of the clinic had been working on bringing their novel idea into existence for 3 years when I met them. My presence filled the void of a psychiatric director, and within months the clinic quickly transformed from a mere idea into a fully functional clinic. The unique strength of this clinic was in creating a space for members of all faith-based communities seeking mental health counseling to potentially access care from professionals of their same faith or, at the very least, from professionals who were rooted in other faith-based traditions. As the clinic opened its doors, a steady stream of Muslim clients from around the Bay Area began to seek me out for counseling.

With encouragement from my mentors, I began to host monthly meetings at Stanford for Muslim mental health professionals who reside in the Bay Area. I had met a handful of Muslim psychiatrists, counselors, social workers, and interested students along the way. It seemed, however, that most of these professionals did not know of each other, and each shared stories of his or her sense of isolation in this field. My goal was to try to bring the few Muslim mental health practitioners scattered across the Bay Area together for networking and support. There had been a previous attempt to accomplish this same goal by a small group of Muslim social workers. After meeting a few times in various coffee shops around town, however, those meetings fizzled out. I wondered if perhaps having consistent meetings in an academic medical setting would help sustain the meetings and give them more credibility.

For the first Bay Area Muslim Mental Health Professionals meeting hosted at Stanford, I reserved a room for about 10 people, double the number of Muslim providers I personally knew. On the day of the first meeting I sat speechless as 20 Muslim mental health professionals crowded into the little room. By the second meeting our number had nearly doubled; word was spreading rapidly. There was a palpable sense of excitement and amazement as the attendees exchanged glances... looks that read, "You're in this field, too?" In introducing themselves, each attendee commented about how he or she was truly shocked at the number of other Muslims in the same field living in the same general area. There was a collective sense of relief in finding one another after individually believing they were the only one trying to provide support for the Muslim community. As the group became better acquainted with one another, networking, mentoring, partnerships, joint research projects and referrals started to take shape organically. These meetings have proven to be the solution to the isolation community-based practitioners were battling and an immense source of support for all of the members involved.

The opportunity to work with the very community I hoped to serve, backed by a strong academic partnership, has proven to be a recipe for success. From a community-based perceptive, my work has been received with appreciation for bringing strong academic credentials down from the perceived "ivory tower" of academia to serve the community. I have found the trust factor and connection with my patients to be stronger by seeing them directly in the community. From an academic perceptive, establishing an "in" with a community that has been dubbed with a "double minority" status would have been nearly impossible to accomplish without community partnerships. My research studies would have been severely limited without community partnerships despite the academic resources available to me at an institution with worldwide fame for its breakthroughs in research. Without community partnerships, it is likely that my research would not have been successful in heralding the accomplishments and advancements it has to date.

Perhaps one of the most fruitful aspects of academic-community partnerships are the opportunities to receive continued mentorship as I further pursue my work with the American Muslim community. In return, the opportunities to mentor the upcoming generation of providers interested in researching and working with the Muslim community seem endless. Recently, I was invited by a mentee to be the keynote speaker for the first ever community-based symposium for the Muslim community specifically dedicated to discussing mental health issues. This successful event was a landmark for our community. At the close of my presentation, one of the most skeptical attendees approached me with tears in his eyes and said, "I have never heard anything like this before. You have completely changed my view about mental illness. May Allah reward you manifold."

My journey thus far has taught me that in order to reach a marginalized community, I must first go directly to the community members and not expect that they will come to me—fancy titles and degrees do little to ameliorate suspicions and fears. Second, I learned that I must speak their language. My community's language is a faith-based language. Being able to draw from my formal Islamic studies and to use my research to educate my clients about our long-lost Islamic heritage and its contributions to the field of mental health have earned me a level of trust no amount of professional training could buy. Third, bridging between medical knowledge, backed by professional training, and Islamic knowledge, backed by formal religious training, has proved to be just the right balance needed to make real and sustainable change in my patients' perspectives. Lastly, the academic-community partnerships created as a result of this work have not only been helpful but imperative in enabling the headway I've made thus far. There is much work yet to do, but I feel confident that things are heading in the right direction, God willing.

Narrative 12
The Intercultural Psychiatric Program at Oregon Health and Science University

James K. Boehnlein, J. David Kinzie, Paul K. Leung, Margaret Cary, Keith Cheng, and Behjat Sedighi

This is the story of a longstanding community-based clinic in Oregon that serves refugees and immigrants from around the world, with the clinical mission of excellence in cross-cultural mental health care and training.

Introduction

It began as the war in Indochina ended. When Saigon fell in 1975, refugees started coming to the United States. Some were sent to Oregon, which traditionally has been receptive to refugees. The first group of refugees was Vietnamese, and among them was a Vietnamese doctor who was admitted to the psychiatry residency program at what was then called the University of Oregon Health Sciences Center in Portland. He and the psychiatry training director, Dr. David Kinzie, began seeing refugee patients in 1978.

Soon refugees from Cambodia and Laos also began to settle in Oregon. A community cultural counseling service as part of refugee support in Portland was started in 1979, and counselors there from Vietnam, Cambodia and Laos referred psychiatric

J.K. Boehnlein, M.D., M.Sc. (✉) • J.D. Kinzie, M.D., F.A.C.Psych.
P.K. Leung, M.D. • B. Sedighi, B.S.
Department of Psychiatry, Oregon Health and Science University, Portland, OR, USA
e-mail: boehnlei@ohsu.edu; kinziej@ohsu.edu; leungpa@ohsu.edu; sedighib@ohsu.edu

M. Cary, M.D., M.P.H. • K. Cheng, M.D.
Division of Child and Adolescent Psychiatry, Department of Psychiatry, Oregon Health and Science University, Portland, OR, USA
e-mail: carym@ohsu.edu; chengk@ohsu.edu

© Springer International Publishing Switzerland 2015
L.W. Roberts et al. (eds.), *Partnerships for Mental Health*,
DOI 10.1007/978-3-319-18884-3_12

patients to our nascent clinic, then called the Indochinese Psychiatric Program. The referred patients were brought by the counselor, who served as an interpreter, with the psychiatrist providing evaluation and treatment. The support of the counseling center ended in 1986, and subsequently the counselors joined our psychiatry department as full-time employees. In those early years of the program when funding was scarce and the future of the program was tenuous, a particularly important central moment occurred that has driven the program and its clinicians ever since.

Central Moment

When we started seeing Cambodians during the first several years, they seemed especially numbed. During a period when continued funding appeared particularly bleak, we told a few of them that we might have to close the clinic. Although their affect and behavior previously had not indicated any particular feelings towards the clinic, that news had a major impact on the patients. They cried and seemed very lost and adrift, acting as if their final support had been taken away from them. Two of them presented to the emergency room with exacerbations of hypertension. The patients later told us, despite their numbness, how much they valued the treatment and how devastating it was to potentially lose this support. We made a decision at that point that we would do everything possible to continuously maintain clinic funding so that we would never have to put our patients through this type of ambiguity that replicated the years of unpredictability and ambiguity during migration and resettlement. Fortunately, we have been able to maintain the clinic for the past 35 years.

Many of the program's original clinicians continue to actively work in administrative and clinical positions. Among the program's original counselors are Kham One Keopraseuth, a senior Laotian counselor who recently retired, and Rath Ben, a senior Cambodian counselor. Dr. Paul Leung began working in the program as a resident in 1981 and has continued through the years as a faculty member, now as professor. Dr. Leung became program director in 1994, a position he has held now for 20 years. Dr. James Boehnlein also began working in the program as a resident in 1983, and continuously has worked in the program as a faculty member since 1987, also now as a professor. Dr. Kinzie, now an emeritus professor, has worked continuously since founding the program in 1978 and has mentored each faculty psychiatrist as they have entered the program.

The model of the program is unique and contributes to its long duration. Each psychiatrist (and faculty member) works with one counselor with one cultural group. The counselor serves as interpreter, case manager, and, with some patients, as a weekly group therapist. Currently the program has 9 part-time psychiatrists and 13 counselors fluent in 16 different languages.

The various cultural groups in the clinic have arrived in the United States following civil war, "ethnic cleansing," and genocide. Refugees come from Bosnia,

Somalia, Ethiopia, Iran, Iraq, Afghanistan, Latin America, Russia, and more recently from Burma and Nepal. As more cultural groups entered the clinic, the name was changed from Indochinese Psychiatric Program to Intercultural Psychiatric Program (IPP).

IPP received a grant from the Office of Refugee Resettlement in 2000 for the treatment of torture survivors. This grant has continued to the present time and has centered a focus on the treatment of torture survivors in some of the program's cultural clinics. From 2002 to 2005, the program received a grant for treatment of traumatized refugee children. This helped to develop the ongoing child psychiatry program within IPP, which will be described in more detail in one of the following sections as an example of IPP's comprehensive treatment.

Research

Academic writing and research has been a major activity at IPP and has contributed to the literature in refugee mental health. We initially published papers on the development of the program, its treatment model, complicated staffing issues, and our initial years of clinical experience [1–5]. Early on we became aware of major depressive disorders among Vietnamese, and with the Vietnamese counseling staff developed the Vietnamese Depression Inventory (VDI) [6], which is still being used in epidemiological studies. When Cambodian refugees arrived, we became aware of the appalling conditions that occurred during the Pol Pot regime and were the first research group to describe posttraumatic stress disorder (PTSD) (which had just been defined in DSM III) among Cambodian refugees [7]. We followed most of the patients after one year and saw much improvement [8]. Unfortunately, most relapsed later and we contributed to the literature showing that PTSD is often a chronic, relapsing disorder in severely traumatized refugees [9]. The central moment described earlier involving the reaction of Cambodian refugees to the tenuous nature of the clinic's survival in its early years strongly influenced our appreciation of the pain suffered by Cambodian survivors of the Pol Pot regime and the direction of our PTSD research over the ensuing decades. This illustrates a recurring pattern in our work—combining research and clinical care to enhance the care of refugee and immigrant patients.

We have continued our clinical research across a number of topics in biological, psychotherapeutic, and social aspects of treatment. It became apparent that many patients, although compliant with appointments, were not taking their prescribed medications. Antidepressant blood levels showed very poor compliance among the Vietnamese and Mien patients and only moderate compliance with Cambodians [10]. This improved among Vietnamese and Cambodians with education, but not among Mien. Group therapy of a special type emphasizing socialization, learning skills, and maintaining cultural events proved to bring improved social functioning among patients [11].

We continued our interest in PTSD and its comorbidities among refugees and identified seven patients with acute psychosis among the initial one hundred Cambodian patients with PTSD [12]. PTSD originally was missed in most non-Cambodian patients until we re-interviewed patients with a formal scale for PTSD and found a highly overlooked prevalence [13].

Over the years it became apparent that all refugee groups had a high prevalence of hypertension and diabetes, and in a study of over 500 of our patients this was further documented [14]. We clearly demonstrated that medical problems represent a significant public health issue for refugees.

A major focus of IPP also has been defining effective treatment for refugees and torture survivors, including pharmacological, psychological, and social interventions. This has included describing effective pharmacological treatment for PTSD hyperarousal symptoms such as nightmares [15–17]. Another important element of our treatment approach has been dealing with ongoing stress of patients and helping staff handle complicated countertransference issues [18, 19]. The most important aspects of treatment are the personal qualities of the therapist [20]. Our clinic has demonstrated that with ethnic counselors, supportive psychotherapy, and medication we can greatly reduce symptoms at follow-up [21].

Clinical Care

We will illustrate the foundation of our clinical care and our comprehensive approach to refugee assessment and treatment first by presenting three clinical vignettes that we have crafted from our experiences in the youth and family program. The vignettes presented here and later in the narrative represent composites of several patients and are typical of individuals in the clinic.

Vignettes

Maahir, a 5-year-old Somali boy, born in Portland, was referred to the youth and family clinic by his mother, due to concerns about his anger. His mother, a refugee from the Somali civil war, receives psychiatric care at the IPP adult clinic. His father is still living in a Kenyan refugee camp.

Mya, a 15-year-old Burmese girl, born in a Thai refugee camp and living in Portland since she was 3 years old, was referred to the clinic by a psychiatric hospital for outpatient care after a suicide attempt. Her parents are not involved with the IPP.

Farzad, a 14-year-old boy born and raised in Afghanistan, was referred to the clinic by his English-as-a-second-language (ESL) teacher, after he had lived in Portland for one year, due to concerns about his distractibility and impulsivity. His mother receives care from the IPP adult clinic.

The Story

The youth and family clinic dovetails with the individual services provided to parents who participate in IPP, further explores the systemic dynamics that promote resilience and contribute to stress, and expands community collaboration through coordination of services with schools, child welfare services, and youth social service programs [22]. Youth and families access the IPP clinic for a diverse range of services including explicit trauma-related symptoms, neurodevelopmental and general psychiatric disorders, and intergenerational cultural conflict. Furthermore, given the sociocentric stance of the families accessing IPP services, attention to family welfare is an expected and integral part of individual care. School staff is always involved to provide collateral information, perspective on the effectiveness of treatment, and additional data on youth function. Primary care providers are included to coordinate health care services. Youth social service agencies are often recruited to provide extra support after school. Finally, Oregon Child Protective Services (CPS) becomes involved when there is concern about the capacity of parents to provide specialized care to children with high needs due to neurodevelopmental disorders, and when there is concern about the appropriateness of parenting practices. While this collaboration with community providers is not unique to the IPP youth and family clinic, the IPP tends to have a greater role in facilitating these collaborations for youth and families due to language, cultural, and educational barriers.

In addition, the generational dynamics of cultural expectations, acculturation differences, parent–child role reversals, and unique trauma experiences complicate the position of the children of refugees.

Because many of these additional specialized services typically do not exist in the families' home countries, and most of them carry significant social stigma, refugee families warrant even stronger collaboration and support than required for average US families. Our youth and family program relies upon existing community programs and services for primary care, academic support, after-school programs, parenting groups, and therapy groups for youth. Because of the trusted relationships formed in IPP, we often know more about the home dynamics, the family stresses, family cultural practices, and the family capabilities than other service providers who have less intimate relationships. Sharing this information is essential for facilitating coordinated and effective support, and linking the perspectives creates solutions. Furthermore, these collaborations can have significant impact on the health of the family. The work with each family exemplifies the reciprocal benefit for both CPS and the family for working collaboratively.

> *"The close collaboration between the therapist and the psychiatrist provides continuity for both the families and community partners. The primary challenge is creating the time to engage in these collaborations."*

> *"Because many of these additional specialized services typically do not exist in the families' home countries, and most of them carry significant social stigma, refugee families warrant even stronger collaboration and support than required for average US families."*

The IPP youth and family clinic, similar to our adult clinics, has two primary providers who collaborate in a multidisciplinary fashion. A therapist who works full-time at the clinic provides case management and individual and family psychotherapy and is the primary person to coordinate care with the family and community providers. The child and adolescent psychiatrist, who works at the clinic part-time, comprehensively evaluates the youth, including exploration of family system dynamics, devises the primary treatment plan, and helps advocate for services. Treatment often involves medication, along with systemic and symptom-targeted psychotherapy, and collaboration with community providers as warranted. The youth and family clinic is the only IPP clinic that is not based on specific cultural groups; therefore, translators are also relied upon as the case manager cannot provide language and cultural translation for all youth and families. A large percentage of the youth speak English, which shifts the majority of the translation challenges to communication with parents rather than the specific clinician/youth therapeutic relationship. The close collaboration between the therapist and the psychiatrist provides continuity for both the families and community partners. The primary challenge is creating the time to engage in these collaborations.

Clinical Vignette: Maahir's Story

Maahir was born in Portland after an uncomplicated pregnancy and birth. His motor skills developed on time, but his language has lagged in both English and Somali. He can identify about half of the letters of the alphabet, can follow simple commands in English and Somali, but rarely speaks, and when he speaks it is in short phrases. Maahir readily and effectively engages in social interactions, responds appropriately in nonverbal ways to social cues, and attends to social interactions. CPS removed his older brother from the home due to the family being unable to provide sufficient care and supervision for his severe neurodevelopmental disorder. Maahir's mother is highly concerned that he will be removed from her care as well, even though she acknowledges his older brother was too much for her to manage as a single parent. Maahir's mother has active PTSD symptoms and is raising her seven other children.

By using a systemic therapy stance, we have learned that Maahir's screaming and aggressive behaviors trigger his mother's PTSD symptoms; she becomes overwhelmed and emotionally reactive and develops headaches. She often has to leave the room or gives curt demands. She is frustrated when Maahir does not follow her bidding. We are concerned that Maahir has an expressive language disorder that leads to frustration about not being fully understood, which explodes in aggressive behaviors. Through addressing the impact of his symptoms on the family, collaborating to devise strategies to support his language development and the treatment of his mother's PTSD symptoms, providing education about both his struggles and PTSD, and teaching additional strategies for communicating with him, we are able to support the healthy function and attachment strengthening of the family while also directly addressing Maahir's needs. Furthermore, through collaboration with CPS, Maahir's mother was invited to join psychiatric appointments with her elder son and his foster family, who are also clients of the IPP youth and family clinic. Maahir's mother was able to demonstrate her own healing and strengthened parenting skills to the foster family, who then advocated for increased parental engagement. This reduced Maahir's mother's suspicion of the foster care program, increased her participation with CPS, supported her relationship with her elder son, and promoted the importance of the family. Thus, with such strategies we are often able to reduce the interventions by CPS. In addition, we have helped facilitate reunification of other clinic families after CPS-mandated separations through collaborations with family support services, school advocates, and law enforcement.

Clinical Vignette: Mya's Story

Mya has been bullied for her appearance, including by other Burmese youth who label her as looking "too Japanese." She now dyes her hair blue, isolates from her family, and restricts her diet. She wants to pursue writing, whereas her parents hope that she will become a physician, lawyer, or engineer. While she feels ostracized by the majority of peers at school, she craves social attachment. This is partly mediated by Mya's attempt to offset the parental role that she assumes at home by navigating cultural barriers for her parents. In addition to providing translation, Mya educates her parents about the school system, the health care system, and Portland teen culture. She sympathizes with their sense of isolation and is protective of their well-being. In addition, Mya discusses how she strives to be loyal to her parents' wishes, appreciating "all they have gone through" to be in the US. Mya also guides her younger brother both in their community cultural practices and integration of their family cultural practices with those of their community. Mya is conflicted about her role, both wanting and not wanting to serve in it.

Mya's suicide attempt was her response to how stuck she feels. Her parents believe that if Mya just listened to them more, she would not be so distressed. Her parents are also strained by their dependence upon Mya. The tensions from this role reversal further distance Mya from her parents during a time when closeness is often sought. In addition, therapeutic interventions must be carefully structured to not alienate either Mya or her parents. For many immigrant and refugee families, the role tensions, parental dependency, and child responsibility result in impairing relational dynamics that must be addressed in order to resolve the psychiatric symptoms. As such, individual-focused psychotherapeutic interventions are insufficient treatment in this clinic, and systemic approaches are the norm. Through the combination of individual and systemic work, Mya has been able to negotiate the tensions of being both an individually focused American teenager and loyal to her familial deference. Both Mya and her parents are attended to without compromising loyalty to either. This has contributed to a willingness of both Mya and her parents to support investigation of alternative school options where Mya might feel more comfortable to explore her identity without compromising her academic goals. Mya also has been freer to accept the dedicated counseling of her school staff, knowing that her parents' position was honored by the IPP staff.

Clinical Vignette: Farzad's Story

Farzad's father was killed during the war in Afghanistan when Farzad was 10 years old. As the eldest son, Farzad started working in a local grocery store to support his mother and two younger siblings. One afternoon Farzad was beaten and stabbed outside of the store. He and his family were eventually granted refugee status and moved to Portland, Oregon. Farzad has had recurrent nightmares since the stabbing and intermittent nightmares since his father's death. He often feels unsettled enough in the morning that he does not eat breakfast. Farzad's birth certificate was mistranslated and initially he was recorded to be 17 years old upon arriving to the United States. Given this, his school peers have been significantly older, and they have taken advantage of Farzad's relative social immaturity. Farzad, who continues to be scared for his safety and fearful of conflict, acquiesces to the older peers' taunts and demands. He also does not ask for help in class, fearing punishment from his teachers. One day Farzad's peers goaded him into a fight, and Farzad was suspended. Without adequate mentoring, positive male role models, and empathy, Farzad's frustration and anxiety have been at risk of escalating into bitterness. Farzad's mother, who also has symptoms of PTSD, is often unable to be fully attentive to Farzad, particularly when he is very upset.

Again, through a systemic, collaborative, and trauma-informed approach, we have advocated for Farzad to be in a developmentally appropriate classroom. We also have facilitated strengthening effective communication between him and his mother. We have helped to untangle which of his impairing symptoms are likely from traumatic stress, which are neurodevelopmental lags in his attention and impulse regulation, and which are interpersonal skills deficits. Finally, we have collaborated with the school to ensure that Farzad is receiving appropriate academic and social support. Although such interventions are time consuming and slow, we have found that fully addressing the complex variables serves to clarify the sources of distress and promotes more resilient healing. Further, these interventions reduce the risk of the youth isolating from their families and engaging in risky or dangerous behaviors.

The IPP youth and family clinic has taught us the importance of validation, a systemic stance, interdisciplinary collaboration, the therapeutic role of advocacy in addition to the social impact, and attending to the complexity of the situation as a means for clarifying the concerns in addition to providing holistic care. As advocacy communicates trust, confidence, and optimism, validation communicates empathy and non-judgment. We are repeatedly reminded that these processes are as therapeutic as the content of our interventions and collaborations. The collaborations are essential for adequate support for the families, brainstorming ideas among providers and families, and strengthening community connections. The systemic stance allows for interventions that encompass both egocentric individual attention and sociocentric family priorities. This supports authentic validation of every family member's perspective, priorities, and experience. It also includes validation of community needs, be it the school's mandate to ensure safety in the classroom, the health clinic's requirement for consistent engagement in care, or the state's expectations for parenting. Such validation fosters engagement, patience, and motivation to participate in the often-challenging coordination and negotiation of care.

As failure to attend to these lessons tends to result in prolonged or less effective care, when treatment is not progressing as anticipated, we slow down and ensure that we are collaborating with the correct service providers, we review our formulations to open space for more complexity, we offer more validation of the relational tensions we have learned about, and we ask what else the families would like us to do for them. While we cannot do all that we would like and all that these families deserve, attempting to understand completely the issues at hand promotes more communication, stronger trust, and greater likelihood of effective support. In addition, identifying the changing of priorities through the treatment process is a systemic measure of change.

As the size of the refugee and immigrant community increases and the funding for social and health services changes, the IPP youth and family clinic identifies different gaps in care, opportunities for care collaboration, and strategies for support. We aim to remain dynamic and flexible to respond to these changes. Thus we are always incorporating the ideas we learn from each other and clients into our work. Finally, we hope that continued community collaborations will result in stronger advocacy for policy revisions both within organizations and at the state level that promote attention to the impact of trauma, acceptance of cultural differences, and coordinated health and social services. In fact, numerous IPP staff members have served as officers in our community's Refugee and Immigrant Consortium, which brings important health and social services information to, and advocates for, refugees and immigrants in Oregon and southwest Washington. The consortium has representatives from a variety of diverse agencies, including the City of Portland, the Oregon Refugee Coordinator's office, Lutheran Community Services, Catholic Charities, and the Immigrant and Refugee Community Organization. Our Socialization Center, which for many years was located in a home leased from a local church, eased the transition to American society by offering language and skills training. For example, while providing culturally diverse food catering to charitable organizations and neighborhood associations, it simultaneously fostered patient skill development and strengthened ties to other community organizations.

Education and Training in IPP

Education and training have been central components of IPP since its inception [23]. Medical students, psychiatry residents, and forensic psychiatry fellows have been the primary groups exposed to the central elements of cross-cultural psychiatric assessment and treatment. Depending on the level of training, education experiences range from primarily observation of faculty clinical work for medical students rotating through the clinic to direct clinical care responsibility for psychiatry residents and fellows.

Medical student observational experiences are offered for OHSU third-year medical students as an option for their half-day/week ambulatory clinic rotations during their 5-week core clerkship and for OHSU and visiting medical students as a 1-month elective fourth-year experience. Students observe various styles of faculty communication with cross-cultural staff and patients, with teaching/mentoring focusing on primary issues such as sensitivity to cultural and family values and beliefs; the impact of historical and political forces on refugee mental health; the relevance of a history of trauma and violence; the impact of rapid cultural change on mental health; and the interface of primary care and mental health in the care of refugees. The overall primary goal for medical student training at IPP is to enhance awareness of the importance of cultural considerations in all of health care, regardless of the eventual career path of the specific student.

Resident rotations in the clinic involve more direct patient care responsibilities. Residents are assigned a caseload of patients under faculty supervision for a period of 6–12 months. That longitudinal patient care responsibility allows residents to observe, assess, and treat complicated mental health problems that are highly influenced by family, social, and community factors. Residents regularly must incorporate into assessment and treatment an awareness of how evolving gender and generational roles during acculturation influence individual identity and family functioning in everyday life and in individuals and families experiencing mental illness. Residents also learn about the important role of social networks in cultural communities, including the impact of both secular and religious networks. The resident learns how to interact with community social service agencies and primary care providers and clinics as a cultural consultant. Also, forensic psychiatry fellows learn how to interact with referring immigration attorneys in their assessment of refugees seeking asylum from political violence or torture.

An important aspect of resident training is experience in the interpersonal elements of cross-cultural care. This includes ongoing interprofessional work within the psychiatrist/case manager dyad. The case manager not only serves as a translator in every clinical session but also is the chief cultural consultant for the resident in their joint care of patients. This provides excellent continuity of care because the case manager has a long-term clinical relationship with that specific group of patients and also is the primary clinician for weekly group therapy for a subset of those patients. In addition, the case manager is frequently the primary team member who extends the team's outreach by making home visits and interacting with community referral sources.

All of these IPP clinical experiences for students, residents, and fellows include the essential experience of being able to examine and discuss cross-cultural transference and countertransference with experienced academic clinicians. These feelings span the spectrum of emotions, from defensive coldness and emotional withdrawal to over-involvement that impairs effective functioning as a clinician. Students and young physicians can be overwhelmed by sadness, frustration, or helplessness. Faculty who have experienced all these feelings over the course of their careers can help guide trainees in learning to recognize and balance their feelings, thereby optimizing clinician mental health and clinical effectiveness. IPP also is an excellent setting for students and residents to witness the central element of trust in patient transference, regardless of cultural group, age, or gender. Dependable, longitudinal treatment in the same clinic, and often with the same clinicians, over decades provides ample evidence of the universal value of trusting relationships and networks in trauma recovery.

This concept is further illustrated by the following clinical vignettes of adult patients in our program, across age and cultural groups. They show the importance of paying close attention to a variety of issues in cultural assessment, including how patients across cultures view age and gender roles, along with the various professional roles of clinicians with whom they are working.

Clinical Vignette

A 35-year-old Vietnamese woman was treated in the clinic for about a year for chronic pain, including headache and backache. At the initial evaluation she said that she was very sad because her husband was killed in Vietnam during the war. As the months progressed she did not improve, and the Vietnamese counselor said that this is a common reaction of Vietnamese women to loss of a husband. Then once, when the counselor was called out of the room, the patient switched over to pretty fair English. Spontaneously, she quickly showed the treating psychiatrist a very scarred leg where her husband had poured boiling water on her. She revealed that he had been quite abusive, and she admitted, in fact, that she was quite glad he was killed, but she could not say that with a Vietnamese female counselor in the room. When the counselor came back, she switched over quickly to talking about her backache, headache, and many other pains. Eventually, over a long period of time, she revealed a more complete marital history in the presence of the counselor.

Clinical Vignette

A 50-year-old African male was known in the community as an angry man. He cussed at people passing by his apartment, and he snarled at people on the street. No one dared go near him because of his anger. He made several clinic appointments but never kept them. When he did finally come for an evaluation it was clear that he did not want to talk about anything in the past. But after the initial, non-confrontational interview, he did open up. He related a wrenching story of rebels coming to his village, lining up the men for execution, and his oldest son stepping in front of him to take a bullet. He had felt intense guilt at this ever since. After that initial session he never talked about it again, but his behavior totally changed. He became polite and gentle in his interactions with others.

IPP Operational Challenges

Operating a comprehensive refugee mental health program that we have described has presented numerous challenges over the years. Many of these challenges will confront almost every community program at one time or another, so some of the most common will be highlighted below.

Financial Challenges

The program relies heavily on Medicaid and Medicare, so it is highly dependent on public funds. We are the primary provider of intercultural services for three local counties. We are subjected to the business practices of the counties, and each of them functions differently. The largest of the three, Multnomah County, holds IPP to the same standards as other mainstream providers but not at the same reimbursement level as those providers. Between 2012 and the end of 2013, this county unilaterally reduced payment by 20 % without prior discussion or room for negotiation. This led to IPP greatly curtailing case management services and counseling to three cultural groups. Referrals from the county were not curtailed, however, and IPP was held responsible for continuing to evaluate new patients within the terms of the original contract.

Over the years, county programs have limited IPP growth by placing a billing cap on delivered services. Regardless of the volume of services provided to IPP clients, the payers capped the amount paid for those services. Even though a cap was placed on reimbursement, an increase in new referrals accepted and services provided was required.

The Affordable Care Act promises new hope in rebalancing the demand for required services with what can be skillfully provided with proper staffing.

Challenges Facing Ethnic Providers

Services can only be reimbursed when rendered by qualified providers. The state of Oregon sets qualification standards through their administrative rules (OARs). The local mental health authority at the county office monitors the application of rules for individual programs such as IPP.

The Oregon administrative rules established two levels of providers: the Qualified Mental Health Professional (QMHP), who is a licensed provider, and the Qualified Mental Health Associate (QMHA), who works under the supervision of a QMHP. The local mental health authority approves the designations upon the submission of the specific employment applications by a program such as IPP.

Variance (waiver) approval for each QMHA and QMHP exists but is rarely issued by the mental health authority of the state. In communities where there is a documented lack of qualified persons, the local mental health authority sometimes will grant designations that do not meet the stated minimum qualifications. IPP over the years has made requests for variance for a number of our ethnic providers serving Bosnian, Somalian, Ethiopian, Iraqi, Afghan, Iranian, Mien, Hmong, Burmese, and Nepalese patients. These are refugee communities in critical need of mental health providers, but it is very difficult to find trained professionals who can meet the minimum qualifications for the QMHA, let alone the QMHP, designation. The variance needs to be renewed annually, with a request submitted to the local mental health authority on behalf of each worker. Over the years the requested variance, when granted, would always come with an increased list of conditions. These would include more supervision by a program QMHP, a demand to return to school to pursue additional education towards a degree, increased level of documentation of supervision and monitoring of the employee, and sometimes even threats to deny payment of services rendered by the employee with variance status.

IPP is the only community agency for referral of refugees and immigrants for mental health assessment and treatment. The caseload of individual providers is two to three times that of providers in mainstream agencies. Providers frequently serve multiple roles, for example, as job counselor, legal aid adviser, community health worker, and housing broker, in addition to their primary role as a mental health provider. Moreover, as a member of the community, the case manager often interacts socially with clients at community events. Although this challenges the case managers in navigating social obligations and professional boundaries within their cultural community, it also provides informal feedback to the clinic about the application and generalization of treatment interventions. Examples include observation of the communication of therapeutic advice, such as medication recommendations discussed by IPP clients with community members not yet ready to come to the IPP. In the Somali community, for example, the recommendation to take omega-3 fatty acid supplements for seasonal affective disorder symptoms and vascular health and to counteract the potential adverse effects of antipsychotic medications has been widely shared. Many Somalis have found omega-3 supplements to be more effective than the antipsychotics and have sustained symptom remission after discontinuation of antipsychotics with maintenance of the omega-3 supplements. Such dissemination of knowledge will, we hope, support the health of the community beyond the direct work with IPP clients. Furthermore, such feedback from the community guides IPP staff to talk with clients about how to share advice and the clinical indications of interventions and to explore thoroughly client understanding and contraindications of interventions. The case managers are essential for enhancing our awareness of the effectiveness of the IPP's clinical care. These additional services are rarely recognized and appreciated by health/mental health/social services authorities in the community.

Finally, since IPP has been so successful in providing effective mental health services to refugees and immigrants despite these challenges, new cultural groups that have been accepted for resettlement in the community routinely are referred to IPP even if there are no established IPP personnel who have cultural and language competency to see the new referrals. This increases pressure on an already burdened system.

Conclusion

It is rare that a community mental health program serving refugees and immigrants is able to survive, much less grow and prosper, over a 35-year period. It is even rarer that it is able to do so with core professional staff members who are able to meet the major clinical, education, and research missions of an academic psychiatry department. As we have discussed, this is not easy because of numerous financial, social, and political challenges occurring over decades that impact program structure and patient care. The IPP, however, shows that this can be done with hard work, dedication, and the constant realization that each of these core missions enriches the other, with the overall primary goal of providing culturally appropriate and comprehensive psychiatric care to refugees and immigrants who have faced great trauma and who continue to face numerous challenges in adjustment and acculturation. The staff's dedication to the mission of the IPP, and the enjoyment of their work, is strongly influenced by observing the healing and growth of refugees who have experienced great loss and pain, as described in the case vignettes. This healing is illustrated in a poetic note of thanks to IPP staff and volunteers, beautifully written by a group of Mien patients after one of their community craft fairs:

> *Your minds are as bright as the sun, which shines down onto the whole world, spreading each one's helpfulness upon us.*
> *Your hearts are as clear as pure water, which enables everyone to see through it.*

References

1. Kinzie JD, Tran KA, Breckenridge A, Bloom JD. An Indochinese refugee psychiatric clinic: culturally accepted treatment approaches. Am J Psychiatry. 1982;139(10):1276–81.
2. Kinzie JD. The establishment of outpatient mental health services for Southeast Asian refugees. In: Williams CL, Westermeyer J, editors. Refugee mental health in resettlement countries. Washington, DC: Hemisphere Publishing Corporation; 1986. p. 217–30.
3. Kinzie JD. Overview of clinical issues in the treatment of Southeast Asian refugees. In: Owan TC, editor. Southeast Asian mental health treatment: prevention, services, training and research. Washington, DC: National Institute of Mental Health; 1985. p. 113–39.
4. Kinzie JD, Manson SM. Five-years' experience with Indochinese refugee patients. J Operational Psychiatry. 1983;14(2):105–11.
5. Kinzie JD. Evaluation and psychotherapy of Indochinese refugee patients. Am J Psychother. 1981;35(2):251–61.
6. Kinzie JD, Manson SM, Vinh DT, Tolan NT, Anh B, Pho TN. Development and validation of a Vietnamese-language depression rating scale. Am J Psychiatry. 1982;139(10):1276–81.
7. Kinzie JD, Fredrickson RH, Ben R, Fleck J, Karls W. Posttraumatic stress disorder among survivors of Cambodian concentration camps. Am J Psychiatry. 1984;141(5):645–50.
8. Boehnlein JK, Kinzie JD, Ben R, Fleck J. One-year follow-up study of posttraumatic stress disorder among survivors of Cambodian concentration camps. Am J Psychiatry. 1985;142(8):956–9.
9. Kinzie JD. The psychiatric effects of massive trauma on Cambodian refugees. In: Wilson JP, Harel Z, Kahana B, editors. Human adaptation to extreme stress: from the Holocaust to Vietnam. New York: Plenum Publishing Corporation; 1988. p. 305–18.

10. Kinzie JD, Leung P, Boehnlein JK, Fleck J. Antidepressant blood levels in Southeast Asians: clinical and cultural implications. J Nerv Ment Dis. 1987;175(8):480–5.
11. Kinzie JD, Leung P, Bui A, Ben R, Keopraseuth KO, Riley C, Fleck J, Ades M. Group therapy with Southeast Asian refugees. Community Ment Health J. 1988;24(2):157–66.
12. Kinzie JD, Boehnlein JK. Post-traumatic psychosis among Cambodian refugees. J Trauma Stress. 1989;2(2):185–98.
13. Kinzie JD, Boehnlein JK, Leung PK, Moore LJ, Riley C, Smith D. The prevalence of post-traumatic stress disorder and its clinical significance among Southeast Asian refugees. Am J Psychiatry. 1990;147(7):913–7.
14. Kinzie JD, Riley C, McFarland B, Hayes M, Boehnlein J, Leung P, Adams G. High prevalence rates of diabetes and hypertension among refugee psychiatric patients. J Nerv Ment Dis. 2008;196(2):108–12.
15. Kinzie JD, Leung P. Clonidine in Cambodian patients with posttraumatic stress disorder. J Nerv Ment Dis. 1989;177(9):546–50.
16. Kinzie JD, Sack RL, Riley CM. The polysomnographic effects of clonidine on sleep disorders in posttraumatic stress disorder: a pilot study with Cambodian patients. J Nerv Ment Dis. 1994;182(10):585–7.
17. Boehnlein JK, Kinzie JD. Pharmacologic reduction of CNS noradrenergic activity in PTSD: the case for clonidine and prazosin. J Psychiatr Pract. 2007;13(2):72–8.
18. Kinzie JD, Boehnlein J. Psychotherapy of the victims of massive violence: countertransference and ethical issues. Am J Psychother. 1993;47(1):90–102.
19. Boehnlein JK, Kinzie JD, Leung PK. Countertransference and ethical principles for treatment of torture survivors. In: Jaranson JM, Popkin MK, editors. Caring for victims of torture. Washington, DC: American Psychiatric Press; 1998. p. 173–84.
20. Kinzie JD. Psychotherapy for massively traumatized refugees: the therapist variable. Am J Psychother. 2001;55(4):475–90.
21. Woticha A, Mohamed H, Kinzie JD, Kinzie JM, Sedighi B. Prospective one-year treatment outcome of tortured refugees: a psychiatric approach. Torture. 2012;22(1):1–10.
22. Kinzie JD, Cheng K, Tsai J, Riley C. Traumatized refugee children: the case for individualized diagnosis and treatment. J Nerv Ment Dis. 2006;194(7):534–7.
23. Boehnlein JK, Leung PK, Kinzie JD. Cross-cultural psychiatric residency training: the Oregon experience. Acad Psychiatry. 2008;32(4):299–305.

Narrative 13
Shared Learning in Community-Academic Partnerships: Addressing the Needs of Schools

Shashank V. Joshi, Roya Ijadi-Maghsoodi, Sarah Estes Merrell, Paul Dunlap, Samantha N. Hartley, and Sheryl Kataoka

This is the story of two partnerships that explores how collaborative relationships develop between local communities and academic researchers, bridge educational needs, and provide mental health services in local school districts.

S.V. Joshi, M.D. (✉)
Department of Psychiatry and Behavioral Sciences,
Stanford University School of Medicine,
Stanford, CA, USA
e-mail: svjoshi@stanford.edu

R. Ijadi-Maghsoodi, M.D.
VA Greater Los Angeles Healthcare System, Health Services Research
and Development Center, Los Angeles, CA, USA
e-mail: rijadimaghsoodi@mednet.ucla.edu

S.E. Merrell, M.A.
St. Ignatius College Preparatory, San Francisco, CA, USA
e-mail: smerrell@siprep.org

P. Dunlap, M.F.A., M.S.
English Department, Henry M. Gunn Senior High School, Palo Alto, CA, USA
e-mail: pdunlap@pausd.org

S.N. Hartley, B.A.
Department of Psychiatry and Behavioral Sciences,
Stanford University School of Medicine, Stanford, CA, USA
e-mail: snh2011@stanford.edu

S. Kataoka, M.D., M.S.H.S.
Division of Child and Adolescent Psychiatry, UCLA Semel Institute, Los Angeles, CA, USA
e-mail: skataoka@ucla.edu

© Springer International Publishing Switzerland 2015
L.W. Roberts et al. (eds.), *Partnerships for Mental Health*,
DOI 10.1007/978-3-319-18884-3_13

Despite national efforts, many youth in the United States do not access mental health services, with only about 21 % of youth in need of a mental health evaluation receiving one [1]. Providing mental health services through schools can reduce access barriers, address stigma, and improve educational outcomes [2, 3]. Providing prevention and early mental health interventions in schools can also be challenging, however, given competing priorities and resources.

From an ecological framework, schools are a crucial primary system to influence a child's social, emotional, and cognitive development. Partnerships between clinician researchers and school communities are important ways to implement existing programs and create new ones that are feasible, sustainable, and acceptable within the school community. This shared partnership, as a community-based participatory process, provides the mutual transfer of expertise in identifying the main concerns, shares decision-making, and gives mutual ownership of the products of the collaboration [4].

In this narrative, we present two examples of school-academic partnerships. The first example describes how clinicians from Stanford University responded to the acute needs of local schools in the San Francisco Bay Area of California following a series of tragic suicides. Through this partnership, academic clinicians assessed the needs of a local community and school district and worked together with community partners to implement an evidence-based suicide prevention program. The second example is from a long-standing partnership developed between the Los Angeles Unified School District and researchers from UCLA and RAND to address a community-defined priority area for services, that of trauma-related mental health symptoms in students as a result of a high prevalence of violence exposure [5]. In both examples, the formation of the partnership, roles of partners, interventions delivered, and lessons learned will be explored.

Example 1: Partnership in Response to Student Suicide

The Partners and What Brought Them Together

As of this writing, suicide accounts for more deaths among 10- to 24-year-olds in the United States than do all natural causes combined [6]. Annually in the United States, about 5–8 % of adolescents attempt suicide, and up to one third of these attempts result in an injury requiring medical intervention [7]. The risk of suicide contagion, a phenomenon defined by the Center for Disease Control and Prevention (CDC) as a process by which exposure to the suicide or suicidal behavior by one or more people influences others to commit or attempt suicide, is especially high in adolescents [8]. Estimates are that more than 100–200 teens die in suicide clusters each year, accounting for about 1–5 % of all teen suicides annually [9, 10]. And suicidal youth may be more "attracted" to death and less able to generate alternatives to suicide when faced with stress, feeling that suicide is a viable (or their only) option [11, 12]. To address this public health problem, school-based suicide prevention programs have become more common as an efficient and cost-effective way to reach adolescents in the context of their daily lives [8].

Two communities in Northern California have recently experienced this phenomenon. Between 2009 and 2010, five Palo Alto teens died by suicide; during a slightly longer time period, four teens at a single school in San Francisco died. Several communities in California have experienced similar losses of their youth to suicide clusters since 2009, and investigations are underway in several of these cities to understand contributing factors [7].

As one school counselor (SM) describes, "The unexpected arrival of a suicide crisis, with the threat of more to come, created an unpredictable climate in our school. Dr. Shashank Joshi, a child and adolescent psychiatrist and Director of School Mental Health at Stanford University, reached out to us after hearing about the suicides in our community and became our academic partner whom I could text, e-mail and talk with, whenever I needed. The partnership meant that we could create a united response to this phenomenon."

Unique Roles in the Partnership: School Counselor and University-Based Psychiatrist

School Counselor: In the first days of our partnership, I (SM) found myself eager to learn while also anxious to be healed (or at least begin the healing process more actively). As a school counselor, philosophically and existentially, I wanted to make sense of the students' decisions to commit suicide, to provide context for the students, and to walk alongside my colleagues. I needed to amass quickly a working knowledge of the science behind suicide and suicide clusters. I found myself fraught with many questions: How do I explain this to the students? What about the parents? How do I care for my colleagues and myself while providing daily outreach and support? How do I ward off compassion fatigue? I knew I needed an action plan that was based on specialized and expert guidance in response to suicide, the prevention of suicide, and how to stop a suicide cluster from growing.

University-based psychiatrist: I (SJ) learned of the suicides at this well-known college preparatory school in our area through a colleague whose wife teaches there. It was clear from the start that, in spite of the best intentions of the administration there and some thought leaders in the parent community, a large obstacle to overcome was the erroneous idea among some senior staff and parents that the school was, in fact, not experiencing a suicide "cluster." Given that several students at one school had taken their lives in a short time period, via similar method, we knew that this community was dealing with what many other San Francisco Bay Area communities had dealt with previously. In spite of citing numerous studies that teaching about depression and suicide risk factors would not increase the risk of more deaths, if done properly, there was still a great deal of stigma that had to be overcome before this school would wholeheartedly embrace the "new normal," that is, that if the school's job was to help all of its students get access to its rich and diverse curriculum, all students had to be "healthy enough to learn." And, we convinced them, mental health is part of health; thus, they should be in the business of both suicide prevention and wellness promotion, starting immediately.

School Counselor: The response to the threat of suicide and contagion was understandably a key part of my role as a school counselor. Dr. Joshi suggested that a plan to assess which students may be at highest risk for self-harm or feeling the most isolated should be among our highest priorities. We began moving through the current crisis and thwarting the real threat of another suicide. Quickly, we had to assess those who were at greatest risk for suicide, rapidly and convincingly referring those students and their parents for diagnoses and care, all while managing the daily paperwork, phone calls, presentations, meetings, and varying student, faculty, and administrative needs.

How the Partnership Identified Needs and Began Delivering Interventions

It was clear that the demands on the counseling department were growing, and they could not do this work alone. Dr. Joshi's team (the academic partners at Stanford University) introduced the school counselors to the Sources of Strength program. This program had shown success in well-designed research around the country at schools that dealt with suicide or had students who were at high risk for suicide attempts [6]. The Stanford team did a presentation for the administration and faculty at this mid-size college preparatory school, as well as for its parent community and Board of Regents, outlining how this program could be the fit the school was looking for, given its focus on peer leader training, campus-wide social messaging activities that focused on the concepts of "Hope, Help, and Strength," and student-adult connections. It could assist the school in characterizing its current climate, assess the connectivity students felt with each other, and describe the ease (or difficulty) with which students felt they could share concerns about their at-risk peers with adults both at school and in the community, if and when they expressed suicidal ideation. The school staff were hopeful that it would help them change the climate of the school and assist them in collecting real-time information from the student body, which would ultimately inform the outreach and prevention program, all in a manner that was statistically sound and proven to work.

One Partner's Perspective

The plan sounded very academic and impressive, but there was still me (SM), feeling strong and committed as a school counselor, yet having an ever-present sense of dread at the prospect of another death around the corner. Getting up each day and going to work was, at times, daunting. I knew that our school was adept at creating connectivity among most students. We provided ample athletic and other extracurricular avenues for building rapport with peers and trusted adults that would lead to natural sources of strength should a student feel in crisis. But yet, what was missing for those students who took their lives? Somehow, their sense of hope was overtaken by their mental experiences with illness, social or family environment, genetic risk, or some combination of these.

It became harder and harder to find compassion satisfaction in our daily work. Instead, symptoms of compassion fatigue and burnout, concepts that the Stanford team had helped us understand better, began to haunt me each day and also plagued the conversations I had with many of my colleagues. We appreciated how, in the face of such difficult daily work following tragedy, some of us move naturally from compassion satisfaction (the pleasure or contentment one derives from one's work) to compassion fatigue (a feeling of tiredness or futility when helping those who are suffering or who have had traumatic stress). As some of us spent more time in the compassion fatigue phase, we also began to notice signs of burnout, such as job dissatisfaction, frustration, irritability, anger, depression, and apathy. First, our Stanford partners convened a grief group with another agency to meet with any faculty and staff in need of support, and what followed were several one-on-one meetings with staff and faculty who felt the need to connect with a mental health provider. This phase was an effective support intervention for front-line staff and helped nurture a feeling of trust, allowing for a sense that we were not alone as staff or as a school or as a community in this struggle. Not long after, a framework for a peer support program was implemented and allowed us to extend our partnership from the faculty and staff to the students. While the Stanford clinicians did not interact directly with the students (we did not need them for this, given our staffing ratios), they were able to provide a "best practice" roadmap and mentorship to the staff, in order to assist the student body.

Since the first days of our partnership, we learned that wellness promotion goes hand-in-hand with suicide prevention. Hence, a comprehensive wellness program was launched and has since become the go-to place for faculty, staff, students, and parents when the need for community referrals or brief clinical assessment is needed. The Wellness Program was in the works before the partnership, but the influx of the suicides accelerated the implementation effort.

Partnership Outcomes

Reflecting on how my work has changed since our partnership, I (SM) have come to appreciate the time I have with each student as sacred. I work with a faster pace and a sharper mind. There is literally a life-and-death aspect that the work takes on with each and every student. Emerging from the crisis were five themes that I continue to frame in all of my student intakes: the state of their family, their health (both mental and physical), their academic progress (or lack thereof), their engagement in the school community, and their social life. I have found that because my time is limited with each student due to his or her protected instructional time, I must remain ever focused on getting to the point each time I have a student contact.

I think that this pressure to be so much to so many could have sunk me if I did not have a strong support system myself in the form of community partnership with clinicians from Stanford. I suppose this is a maturation of my school-counseling role that is understandable, given the cluster of suicides that has informed my work and provided me with school mental health mentors. I also rely more and more on a network of students I have established relationships with, so that they can inform me of students they are aware of who may need counseling support. I also work from the understanding that I need to take care of myself if I am to remain effective and strong. Self-care continues to be a real focus for both me and for my colleagues.

The Partnership and the Work

Collaborating with the school mental health team at Stanford is evolving and always seems to be in sync with the needs of the core counseling staff working on suicide prevention, wellness promotion, and creative outreach efforts. Mostly, the Stanford partners provide expert guidance and continual (twice yearly) assessment of how our work has affected the students' perceptions of help-seeking behavior, what barriers exist to accessing help, and the availability of adult support. The team of school counselors then works with students to identify how to make accessing support more realistic.

I (SM) am part of a core group of four counselors who make up the outreach team and work directly with the students. When we began the Sources of Strength project, students were appointed by a faculty of 130 to ensure a cross section of students in order to have a peer leader group size that was as diverse as possible, across class, social, racial, and ethnic lines. After our students were identified, we brainstormed how to identify "who we are" and what we wanted to achieve.

Lessons Learned and Future Directions for the Partnership

Social messaging campaigns are designed to encourage students to feel less shame about mental health concerns and more connectivity within the school campus and community at large. Our partnership with the Stanford team has allowed us to have a real-time link to experts and to be part of a team of allies who join us in understanding and addressing the complex emotions and behaviors of some of our students. In this partnership, I (SM) have found listening ears, a "no judgment" atmosphere and ongoing support of my direct service work. As a school counselor, just knowing that there are expert clinicians working with me, I am more eager and energized to continue the work and find that I can more readily ward off compassion fatigue.

When we first met our relationship was similar to that of a teacher and student or doctor and patient. In many ways the partnership continues to be a nurturing and evolving dynamic as our school climate changes (per the data) and as we change. The expert theory we rely on to guide our next moves are informed by our now longstanding work together. In other words, we don't need to pick up a book or reach out for technical assistance; rather, technical assistance is alongside us each day, a reciprocal approach to direct service and academic knowledge.

With the support and partnership of a prestigious university and experts in the field of suicide prevention, I believe our school counseling team has the opportunity to engage students in creative programing that increases student involvement because it is affiliated with academic research. The students are eager to affect the suicide prevention knowledge base and this eagerness energizes the peer outreach activities that students engage in. The challenge before us was, "How do we make suicide prevention relevant and compelling to all students?" And, "How do we find connectivity through experiences that can isolate teens from one another due to shame or the social withdrawal that can accompany many mental health disorders?"

It has taken direct contact with adults who are both approachable and creative for the word to spread that seeking help for a distressed peer is crucial and can be lifesaving. The once secretive dynamic that keeps youth and adults separated when it comes to mental health issues can in fact be redesigned, replaced with an ongoing invitation for youth to share with trusted adults. The secretive dynamic must constantly be chipped away by campaigns that encourage help-seeking behavior, and we have begun to do that on our campus. After just 5 months of "hope, help, and strength" messaging, we have changed the norm so

> *"Teens struggling with depression, anxiety, eating disorders, substance abuse, and self-harm are not new to our school community. What is unique is that they are being invited to talk about these once-taboo topics. In order to prevent the isolation and reduce the stigma associated with these conditions, our work includes meeting regularly to establish that we are a group of trusted adults who are committing ourselves to them."*

that teens no longer feel that getting help for a severely distressed friend is getting them *into* trouble but, rather, is getting them *out of* trouble. The research findings from the first year showed there were significantly more trusted adult–student relationships in comparison with the baseline, and almost twice as many students could name trusted adults they would go to on campus than at the baseline. These findings have continued in years 2 and 3, and those students who have shown the most benefit are the ones at highest risk for suicide attempts.

Teens struggling with depression, anxiety, eating disorders, substance abuse, and self-harm are not new to our school community. What is unique is that they are being invited to talk about these once-taboo topics. In order to prevent the isolation and reduce the stigma associated with these conditions, our work includes meeting regularly to establish that we are a group of trusted adults who are committing ourselves to them. The very act of regularly meeting to discuss what "we don't usually talk about" is edgy. This real and honest approach to taboo subjects has proven to be very appealing to teens.

From the vantage point of the academic partner, we have appreciated how important it is to avoid a one-size-fits—all approach to this work, as individual school districts and school communities have unique histories and subcultures that must be understood before any sort of intervention is undertaken, even for basic grief support following a school tragedy. Still, some wise-minded guidelines regarding process variables are helpful to remember [8, 13–15], especially in the face of such tragic events as a suicide of someone in the school community.

The "3 Rs" of school consultation [15] include the *relationships* that need to be cultivated and fostered, the *recognition* of human motivation during an important or sensitive time, and the *responses* to challenges. For us as the academic partner, each "face time contact" with administration was an opportunity to improve the school ethos and its response to not only those in greatest need but also the system as a whole. We have been very mindful of these "3 Rs."

First, our academic partner strengthens the relationships of professionals allied around students, parents, and the greater school community, building bridges among them. This partnership among parents, staff, and therapists for school mental health has been termed *the supporting alliance in school mental health* and has been described previously [16].

Second, the academic partner can foster recognition of human motivation and the resistance that may impede healthy changes in the case of suicide prevention. Guiding principles include determining the wishes and motives of the student, parent, teacher, and administrator and dismantling resistance to change. We acknowledged (even normalized) that the reluctance to embark on universal suicide prevention strategies often stems from a place of fear (e.g., that such programs may "plant" the idea of suicide not only in vulnerable youth but also in those who had not considered suicide previously) in order to correct this misconception [17, 18].

Third, as the academic partner, we can help the staff create responses to challenges. Guiding principles include providing staff new skills to reach and teach distressed students and finding common goals to unite students in the school, to reach parents in the community (especially thought leaders in the parent-teacher association), and to determine the developmental steps toward shared goals [15].

Finally, as academic-school consultant partners, we can leverage the trust we have built with school administration and school district leadership to advocate for school climate and other structural changes that have an emerging research base in support of youth mental health. These include later school start times to improve total sleep [19]; detailed self-study into the sources of major and daily stressful life events for youth [20], such as severe academic stress in communities where youth may see themselves as being evaluated solely in terms of their academic performance and the pressure to excel is an important measure of their success in school [21]; and the adoption of formal suicide prevention policies with administrative regulations by local school boards [22]. The aforementioned empowering principles allow therapeutic skills used in individual and family therapies to provide strategies that can assist education professionals, students, and the larger school community simultaneously [8].

An Educator's Perspective: Reach Out, Care, Know

Two students approached me (PD) with the desire and rough plans to share the strength they found in each other ("rocks," they called themselves), in the wake of five suicides of members of our student body. Knowing both how students more readily share personal struggles with peers before adults and how they would need an adult advisor to help with logistics, they asked me to be their advisor. Sources of Strength and Dr. Joshi's team approached us with the idea of a newly formed peer support group, ROCK (Reach Out, Care, Know), to partner with them and use their evidence-based peer leader training practices as a natural fit.

Over 60 students and 20 faculty members participated in the first training. When it came to follow-up meetings, the group was enthusiastic but increasingly small. Clearly harmonious with the school mission, the program's placement in school structure and administrative priorities was unclear. As is true with many worthy activities, ROCK and Sources of Strength relied on the commitment of students who were already very busy. Rather than a schoolwide movement, ROCK was perceived by some as my project, something antithetical to our goal.

Dr. Joshi and the project director, Sami Hartley, returned to a staff meeting to present initial findings and possible follow-up steps and met with us several other times to discuss vision and effectiveness with the student group. More recently, they met with administrators and TOSAs (Teachers on Special Assignment) to share ideas about what Sources of Strength could look like at our high school moving forward. These conversations clarified ways that TOSAs could support the work, including the schoolwide logistical planning that is challenging for a single full-time teacher.

Not surprisingly, the issues have personally touched many students who are drawn to specific work regarding emotional well-being and suicide prevention. Partnering with the Stanford team has been particularly helpful in discussing some specific students, including some of the student leaders. Not a professional in these topics, I have had to do what I tell students to do: Reach out to professionals when issues transcend my training. After 4 years of relative health (and no student deaths), we lost two school community members this fall. The ROCK student leaders received more attention, but they also felt worried. Some felt as if the work they were doing was futile. If spending countless hours committed to promoting connection on campus could not prevent suicides, what was it all worth? I met with them regularly, twice with our new principal, to convey deeper structural support and remind them of the success of the previous 4 years. I required each student leader to make an appointment with a counselor of some sort, whether on campus or in the community at large. Initially reluctant, they did so and were glad.

Active partnership with both the school and academic communities is essential for these students to feel strong enough to address issues of resilience and courageous enough to wear T-shirts exhorting others to "Talk To Me." This takes committed students and faculty who do not need to have all (or any of) the answers, but they need the support of the community-academic partnership and, above all, time.

Example 2: Partnership to Meet the Needs
of Students Exposed to Violence

The Partners and What Brought Them Together

"Why are you talking to me about suicide? It is violence exposure that is the problem for our students!" This exclamation by a Los Angeles Unified School District (LAUSD) teacher during a suicide prevention focus group summed up the identified and pervasive problem of community violence affecting many students and teachers in this large urban school district. As the second largest school district in the country, LAUSD serves a predominantly poor population, with over three quarters of students qualifying for free or reduced lunch and the vast majority of students being of an ethnic minority background, including 74 % who are Latino.

Over 15 years ago, clinician-researchers from UCLA and RAND and community partners from the LAUSD's mental health unit and the director at the time, Dr. Marleen Wong, began a school community-research partnership [23]. Dr. Wong had been instrumental in developing the district's crisis teams, a model for the nation, but recognized the need to also deliver broader mental health services to prevent these crises. At the time that this partnership began, she had additional district funding to support an expansion of school mental health services for new immigrant students, those in the country 3 years or less, who often had experienced multiple traumas in their home country, during the immigration process, and in their new Los Angeles neighborhoods and who were at risk for poor academic achievement and dropout. She sought a partnership with an expert in treatment of post-traumatic stress disorder at RAND and had the vision to simultaneously engage researchers at UCLA and RAND to evaluate those services to ensure that the end product went beyond "feel good therapy" and was shown to improve outcomes for students.

Some of the research partners began this collaboration while still in research training as part of the UCLA Robert Wood Johnson Clinical Scholars Program, with support from senior faculty on methods in community partnership, evaluation, and intervention development. Although courses in biostatistics and research design were important, Dr. Wong's "classroom" in the schools and hearing the concerns of principals and experiences of her large staff of psychiatric social workers, as well as students and parents, were some of the most meaningful lessons in conducting community partnered research. Dr. Wong shared her experiences of "getting in the door" with schools by responding to the immediate needs of a school whether during a school shooting or suicide attempt or other crises. Through these incidents, the relevance for mental health services became more evident to principals and school staff. In this large urban school district, one priority for the mental health team has been addressing the effects of community violence and providing early intervention to improve students' ability to participate in the educational curriculum.

Unique Roles in the Partnership

Within the constraints of the school system, the school partners identified the pervasive exposure to trauma and violence as their priority. Research partners developed an intervention protocol based on proven intervention elements and suggested evaluation designs. Although the best-proven treatment protocols for adults consisted of 90-minute individual sessions delivered by expert research psychologists, the school partners wanted to create a program that could be delivered by their existing social work staff in the 45 minutes of a typical school therapy session, and utilizing a group modality to serve more students. A flexible intervention model that could be modified for different cultures, languages, and neighborhoods was also critical in a district where more than 52 languages are spoken.

In reviewing options for the evaluation, research partners presented several options for standardized assessment measures, comparison groups, and research designs. Instead of lengthy evaluation questionnaires and intensive diagnostic assessments, school partners opted for brief screening surveys that school clinicians could administer and were not excessively burdensome to the students, parents, and teachers. Not only were mental health symptoms of posttraumatic stress and depression measured, but school partners also emphasized the importance of measuring educational outcomes, given the accountability of school mental health services to addressing the educational mission of schools. School partners also preferred a waitlist comparison design instead of a control group that only included an outside referral, given that few students accessed off-campus treatment when referred.

How the Partnership Identified Needs and Delivered an Intervention

To confirm their speculation that violence exposure was pervasive in this district, the school district surveyed over 28,000 sixth-grade students about their exposure to violence. In this community-research partnered study, investigators found that 40 % of these students reported knife or gun violence in the past 12 months, life-threatening violence that resulted in direct victimization of or witnessing by students [24]. School partners linked this survey data to school administrative data that illustrated the relationship between types of exposure to violence and associations with suspensions and absenteeism.

The Cognitive Behavioral Intervention for Trauma in Schools (CBITS) [25] developed by this school community-research partnership was one that "fit" within the context of schools and was based on the best evidence for treating trauma-related mental health problems in youth [26]. As seen in Fig. 13.1, the community-research partnership was key to each phase of intervention development and implementation. Clinician-researchers partnered with the school social workers in conducting a randomized controlled trial, first piloting the intervention through an iterative process

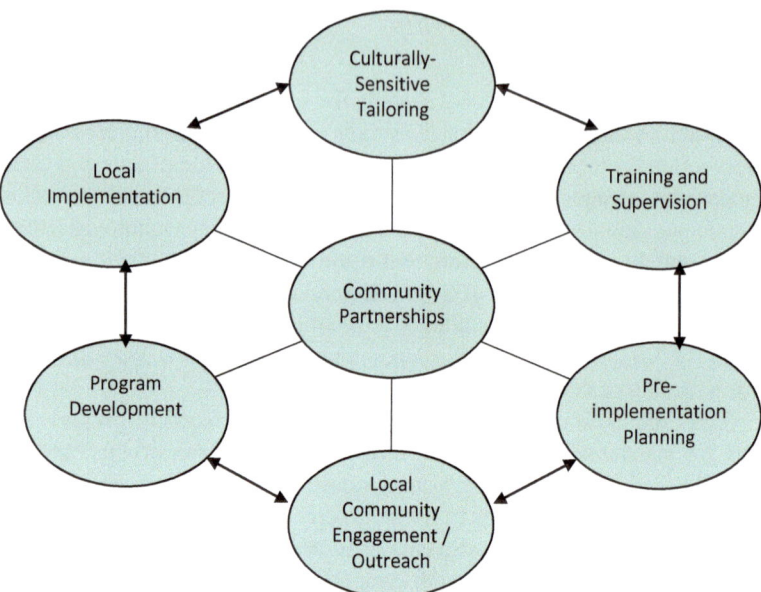

Fig. 13.1 Model for using community partnerships to provide culturally sensitive, evidence-based treatment. Reprinted from J Am Acad Child Adolesc Psychiatry, 47/8, Ngo V, Langley A, Kataoka SH, Nadeem E, Escudero P, Stein BD: Providing evidence-based practice to ethnically diverse youths: examples from the Cognitive Behavioral Intervention for Trauma in Schools (CBITS) program, pages 858–62, Copyright 2008, with permission from the American Academy of Child and Adolescent Psychiatry

of quality improvement. These district school social workers identified which sessions required more time to deliver, provided examples of alternative ways to implement, and created whole toolkits for easier implementation which included form letters to parents and principals and calendar examples of fitting CBITS into the school calendar (avoiding state testing and scheduled breaks), all of which allowed for shared resources and less duplication of effort in delivering this intervention for the first time.

CBITS was the first effectiveness trial of a school-based trauma intervention to demonstrate in a randomized controlled trial improved depression and symptoms of posttraumatic stress disorder (PTSD) [5, 27]. CBITS is delivered in 10 group-based sessions and focuses on teaching students core cognitive-behavior skills, including relaxation, problem-solving, and cognitive restructuring. A priority outcome for schools has also been academic outcomes, and in preliminary findings, CBITS appears to improve reading and math grades [28]. CBITS has been now widely disseminated across the United States and internationally, and it is identified as an evidence-based treatment nationally as well as in Los Angeles County and California, which allows for billing of this service and a path to sustainability.

Partnership Outcomes

As discovered through this partnership, implementation of school mental health interventions can be challenging, given that this is a non-mental health system [29]. Screening for PTSD symptoms on campus has been recognized by school partners as a key component of CBITS implementation, because many students otherwise go undetected. School clinicians would hear from students who had experienced violence yet had no adult in their lives who was aware of the trauma or its impact on the student. Obtaining parental consent for a school screening can present major challenges, however, including misperceptions and fears about the intent of the questions or views of violence exposure as "normal in our community." Broad educational outreach about the impact of trauma on youth and the effects of trauma on school success has been a major effort of our school community-research partnership. As a result, several innovative solutions to "getting the word out" were created: a jointly made video of students and school community members talking about the effects of trauma on youth (now also available in Spanish), partnering with faith organizations and lay health promoters to outreach to the faith community [30], and students themselves developing poetry readings to share with their school community how they have moved forward toward a path to wellness.

Another major barrier to implementing treatments in schools is the lack of infrastructure that frequently exists in a specialty mental health center to support training and delivery of evidence-based treatments. Frequently school mental health clinicians have few clinical colleagues on campus with whom to consult when cases present challenges. As our school partners and sites across the country were faced with these challenges, we partnered with our school colleagues in developing online resources that can be readily accessed. At CBITSprogram.org, school-based clinicians can access and post adaptations and tools that have been developed in the field to facilitate implementation. An online training and "quick tips" and "ask the expert" resources have been co-developed between research clinicians and school partners to make tools relevant for school communities and to support dissemination efforts [31]. From development, to evaluation, to implementation and dissemination, this CBITS school community-research partnership has guided program development and research efforts that respond to the real needs of communities.

Lessons Learned and Future Directions for the Partnership

This school community-research partnership has resulted in the CBITS intervention and others being developed and disseminated nationally and internationally. The research evidence has led to CBITS being listed in local and national registries of evidence-based practices, allowing for billing and sustainment of the intervention delivery. The partnership itself has sustained through multiple grants to support the community efforts, mainly through funding from the Substance Abuse and Mental Health Services Administration and National Institute of Health support for research. Finally, the responsiveness of our partnered team to the real needs of "on the ground" clinicians has resulted in implementation tools to improve dissemination. From this work, one direction that our partnership has been taking is a broader "Trauma-Informed School" approach, with attention to a school climate that supports students who have experienced trauma, resources for teachers and school staff who have experienced primary and secondary traumatic stress, and primary prevention in classrooms that teach students better communication and coping skills in addition to early and intensive interventions for those students with PTSD.

Another lesson learned through these school community-academic partnerships with LAUSD has been the generative role of continuing to train clinicians and researchers in community partnerships. Having clinicians-in-training learn experientially how academic institutions can effectively partner with school communities will prepare our future workforce to better understand this model of a two-way shared knowledge exchange. Creating an environment in which postdoctoral fellows and junior researchers can become involved in established partnership projects is critical for a research agenda that includes the encouragement of community partnered research to decrease disparities and improve access to mental health care for all students. RIM, a trainee who conducted focus groups with students to understand the barriers to seeking mental health care and ways to improve engagement in mental health services through school-based health centers, summarizes her experiences in this way:

In my training as a child psychiatrist, I constantly strive to give something to my patients in the therapy sessions. A validation of their experience, an insight to take with them, sometimes just a calm place to play and be heard, even if they do not want to speak in words. Yet in the focus groups, the students gave us much more than we could offer them. The groups were not a question-and-answer session, nor a therapy group. They were an invitation into the students' world, a place where they answered honestly and openly. They spoke about stress, not just stress from grades or tests, but from their daily lives, "relationships…abuse…family abuse…family problems." They spoke about how students kept things inside, due to embarrassment, fear of being judged, or secrets being exposed. They described a need for connection, trust, and, most of all, for someone to understand their experiences. What they told us not only informed our research, and ultimately the district's services, but also impacted my clinical work. I found myself listening differently with my patients and inquiring more about their environments and about the quality of their relationships with teachers and staff at school.

We all felt the need to give something back to the students who had so poignantly affected us. Without the barrier of the white coat or the formality of a clinic evaluation, we took on a different role with the students, distinct from our role of researcher or clinician. At the end of the focus groups, we turned off the recorders and opened up time for questions they had for us. Many eagerly asked about different colleges, if they could handle the workload, and what our experiences had been. At that moment, we became mentors and gave encouragement and support to these LAUSD students.

The students transformed our way of thinking about their struggles, about the schools, and about their lives. In the space of the group, when the students spoke to each other, and validated one another, the hope is that they also gained something. Group dialogue about one's community has the potential to facilitate self-reflection, understanding of barriers, and, I hope, plant seeds of empowerment for change. This power of reflective knowledge has been described as the "power of competence, connection, and confidence" [32].

Conclusion

Community-academic partnerships provide essential two-way learning, not only by supporting the community partner but also by informing and transforming the academic researcher. As demonstrated by the two examples in this narrative, school-academic partnerships can build on the strengths of communities and together create unique solutions to urgent needs. In this era of health care reform, identifying how social determinants of mental health such as education and needs of the community can be addressed, while at the same time bolstering the strength of the community and partnering with community members to improve health in a mutual process, will grow ever more important.

Acknowledgements   This work was supported by SAMHSA SM59285 (Wong) and the Office of Academic Affiliations through the VA Advanced Fellowship Program in Women's Health (Ijadi-Maghsoodi). The authors also thank Dr. Marleen Wong for her leadership and partnership, the staff and students of St. Ignatius College Preparatory High School, Henry M. Gunn High School, and the Los Angeles Unified School District.

References

1. Kataoka SH, Zhang L, Wells KB. Unmet need for mental health care among U.S. children: variation by ethnicity and insurance status. Am J Psychiatry. 2002;159(9):1548–55.
2. Keeton V, Soleimanpour S, Brindis CD. School-based health centers in an era of health care reform: building on history. Curr Probl Pediatr Adolesc Health Care. 2012;42(6):132–56.
3. Walker SC, Kerns SEU, Lyon AR, Bruns EJ, Cosgrove TJ. Impact of school-based health center use on academic outcomes. J Adolesc Health. 2010;46:251–7.
4. Viswanathan M, Ammerman A, Eng E, Garlehner G, Lohr KN, Griffith D. Community-based participatory research: assessing the evidence. Evid Rep Technol Assess (Summ). 2004;(99):1–8.
5. Kataoka SH, Stein BD, Jaycox LH, Wong M, Escudero P, Tu W. A school-based mental health program for traumatized Latino immigrant children. J Am Acad Child Adolesc Psychiatry. 2003;42(3):311–8.
6. Wyman PA, Brown CH, LoMurray M, Schmeelk-Cone K, Petrova M, Yu Q, et al. An outcome evaluation of the sources of strength suicide prevention program delivered by adolescent peer leaders in high schools. Am J Public Health. 2010;100(9):1653–61.
7. Centers for Disease Control. Youth Risk Behavior Surveillance, United States 2013; Surveillance Summaries. 63(4) June 13, 2014; Accessed 9/1/14.
8. Joshi SV, Hartley SN, Kessler M, Barstead M. School-based suicide prevention: content, process, and the role of trusted adults and peers. Child Adolesc Psychiatr Clin N Am. 2015;24:353–70.
9. Gould MS, Wallenstein S, Kleinman MH, O'Carroll P, Mercy J. Suicide clusters: an examination of age-specific effects. Am J Public Health. 1990;80(2):211–2.
10. Hacker K, Collins J, Gross-Young L, Almeida S, Burke N. Coping with youth suicide and overdose: one community's efforts to investigate, intervene, and prevent suicide contagion. Crisis. 2008;29(2):86–95.

11. Brent DA. Preventing youth suicide: time to ask how. J Am Acad Child Adolesc Psychiatry. 2011;50(8):738–40.
12. Orbach I, Rosenheim E, Hary E. Some aspects of cognitive functioning in suicidal children. J Am Acad Child Adolesc Psychiatry. 1987;26:181–5.
13. Weist MD, Lowie JA, Flaherty LT, Pruitt D. Collaboration among the education, mental health, and public health systems to promote youth mental health. Psychiatr Serv. 2001;52(10):1348–51.
14. Waxman RP, Weist MD, Benson DM. Toward collaboration in the growing education-mental health interface. Clin Psychol Rev. 1999;19(2):239–53.
15. Bostic JQ, Rauch PK. The 3 R's of school consultation. J Am Acad Child Adolesc Psychiatry. 1999;38(3):339–41.
16. Feinstein NF, Fielding K, Udvari-Solner A, Joshi SV. The supporting alliance in child and adolescent treatment: enhancing collaboration between therapists, parents and teachers. Am J Psychother. 2009;63(4):319–44.
17. Gould MS, Greenberg T, Velting DM, Shaffer D. Youth suicide risk and preventive interventions: a review of the past 10 years. J Am Acad Child Adolesc Psychiatry. 2003;42(4):386–405.
18. Gould MS, Marrocco FA, Kleinman M, Thomas JG, Mostkoff K, Cote J, et al. Evaluating iatrogenic risk of youth suicide screening programs: a randomized controlled trial. JAMA. 2005;293(13):1635–43.
19. American Academy of Pediatrics [Adolescent Sleep Working Group, Committee on Adolescence, and Council on School Health]. School start times for adolescents. Pediatrics. 2014;134:642–9.
20. Wagner BM, Cole RE, Schwartzman P. Psychosocial correlates of suicide attempts among junior and senior high school youth. Suicide Life Threat Behav. 1995;25(3):358–72.
21. Ang RP, Huan VS. Relationship between academic stress and suicidal ideation: testing for depression as a mediator using multiple regression. Child Psychiatry Hum Dev. 2006;37: 133–43.
22. Joshi SV, Hartley SN, Lenoir L, Ojakian M. A comprehensive suicide prevention toolkit (166 pages). Palo Alto, CA: PAUSD Press; 2013.
23. Wong M. Commentary: building partnerships between schools and academic partners to achieve health related research agenda. Ethn Dis. 2006;16(1 Suppl 1):S149–53.
24. Ramirez M, Wu Y, Kataoka S, Wong M, Yang J, Peek-Asa C. Youth violence across multiple dimensions: a study of violence, absenteeism, and suspensions among middle school children. J Pediatr. 2012;161(3), 542–6. e542.
25. Jaycox LH. Cognitive-behavioral intervention for trauma in schools. Longmont, CO: Sopris West Educational Services; 2003.
26. Stein BD, Kataoka SH, Jaycox LH, Wong M, Fink A, Escudero P. Theoretical basis and program design of a school-based mental health intervention for traumatized immigrant children: a collaborative research partnership. J Behav Health Serv Res. 2002;29(3):318–26.
27. Stein BD, Jaycox LH, Kataoka SH, Wong M, Tu W, Elliott MN. A mental health intervention for school children exposed to violence: a randomized controlled trial. JAMA. 2003;290(5): 603–11.
28. Kataoka SH, Jaycox LH, Wong M, Nadeem E, Langley A, Tang L. Effects on school outcomes in low-income minority youth: preliminary findings from a community-partnered study of a school trauma intervention. Ethn Dis. 2011;21:S1.
29. Langley AK, Nadeem E, Kataoka SH, Stein BD, Jaycox LH. Evidence-based mental health programs in schools: barriers and facilitators of successful implementation. School Ment Health. 2010;2:105–13.
30. Kataoka SH, Fuentes S, O'Donoghue VP, Castillo-Campos P, Bonilla A, Halsey K. A community participatory research partnership: the development of a faith-based intervention for children exposed to violence. Ethn Dis. 2006;16(1 Suppl 1):S89–97.
31. Vona P, Wilmoth P, Jaycox LH, McMillen JS, Kataoka SH, Wong M. A web-based platform to support an evidence-based mental health intervention: lessons from the CBITS web site. Psychiatr Serv. 2014;65(11):1381–4.
32. Park P. Knowledge and participatory research. In: Reason P, Bradbury H, editors. Handbook of action research: participative inquiry and practice (Concise ed.). Thousand Oaks, CA: Sage; 2006. p. 83–93.

Narrative 14
The Earthquake

Jayne E. Fleming and Daryn Reicherter

This is the story of how four doctors, a global law firm, and three human rights lawyers launched a humanitarian parole project in response to the catastrophic impact of an earthquake in Haiti in 2010.

On January 12, 2010, there was a magnitude 7.0 earthquake in Haiti. It was centered in the city of Leogane but cut a much wider path of destruction. Huge areas of Port au Prince and the surrounding cities were destroyed. Over a half million buildings collapsed, including 250,000 homes, 30,000 businesses, 4000 schools, the Presidential Palace, the Port au Prince Cathedral, the Palace of Justice, churches, hospitals, clinics and the national penitentiary. All but one government building was destroyed, as well as 60 % of hospitals and 80 % of schools.

The earthquake was on a Tuesday, just before 5:00 pm. The time of day is meaningful for two reasons. First, it was late enough that many school-aged children were not at their desks when their schools caved in. Second, it was early enough that many adults were at work when their offices and shops collapsed. Many children escaped death; many adults did not. Nobody knows how many Haitians were buried under rubble. Officials estimate that more than 250,000 people died and more than

J.E. Fleming, J.D. (✉)
Firm Reed Smith LLP, New York, NY, USA
e-mail: jfleming@reedsmith.com

D. Reicherter, M.D.
Department of Psychiatry and Behavioral Sciences,
Stanford University School of Medicine, Stanford, CA, USA
e-mail: reichertermd@yahoo.com

© Springer International Publishing Switzerland 2015
L.W. Roberts et al. (eds.), *Partnerships for Mental Health*,
DOI 10.1007/978-3-319-18884-3_14

200,000 children became orphans. Over a million people became homeless. Port au Prince became a labyrinth of camps spilling onto streets, filling public spaces, and climbing the hills surrounding the capital. There were over a thousand camps.

The day after the disaster, military troops, aid workers, diplomats, and Good Samaritans began arriving in Port au Prince. Dozens of foreign journalists descended on the capital to broadcast the tragic images: a man searching through rubble for a missing relative; a mother cradling the body of a dead child; an old woman bent in prayer before a collapsed church. Some saw this endless coverage as an assault on the privacy of victims. Others saw it as key to mobilizing a global relief effort.

A month after the disaster, four Stanford doctors, a global law firm (Reed Smith LLP), and three human rights lawyers teamed up to send a delegation to Haiti. All of the team members had worked with refugees and displaced populations from around the world; all had studied the intersections between extreme poverty, international crisis, and human rights abuses. The goal was to evaluate the impact of the earthquake through a human rights lens and ask whether the Haitian government, the United Nations (UN), and non-governmental organizations (NGOs) were living up to their duty to protect displaced people. A related goal was to identify Haitians who might qualify for evacuation to the United States on the basis of extraordinary circumstances like a life-threatening medical problem or other threat of serious harm. Four years and some 30 trips later, the team evacuated 60 vulnerable women and children from Haiti to the United States and Canada. This is how we did it.

Arrival

We arrived in Haiti in early March 2010. As we approached the airport to land, we could see a hospital ship and at least 20 smaller ships anchored off the coast of Port au Prince. A line of cargo planes on the tarmac grew bigger as we approached the runway. We could see thousands of tents covered with blue and orange plastic tarps surrounding the airport, covering flat brown fields and climbing the hills.

A Haitian man named Charles[1] met us at the airport. He worked as a fixer for foreign journalists, part of a valuable cadre of trilingual interpreters who doubled as drivers. He was also a law student and prison rights activist. We had hired him to protect us, drive us, and interpret for us. He would soon become an indispensable member of our team.

After leaving the airport, we drove to downtown Port au Prince. Nearly every building was either badly damaged or destroyed. The streets were filled with rubble. People had set up tents on the sides of roads, on top of collapsed buildings, and in front of stores with gaping holes. Many streets were so crowded with tents they were impassable. It was like a world turned inside out, with everyone living under the sky, and all of the buildings turned upside down.

---

[1] Names have been changed to protect the identities of the individuals described in the narrative.

The pulse of activities in the streets seemed chaotic but had a rhythm, like a drumbeat or a dance. There were women grilling chicken on the side of the road. The women were also selling raw meat, and swarms of flies infected the meat like living measles. There were hundreds of women carrying things on their heads—baskets of avocados, buckets of produce, cooking pots, tubs of charcoal, housewares, cookware, baskets of live chickens drooping under the tropical heat. Some women carried babies in their arms, shielding their faces from clouds of black exhaust and dirt and ash. Some girls held hands as they walked; others sat on the edge of the roadside, staring as we passed.

It was a harsh and extraordinary scene. We wanted to take pictures but felt unsure. "Go ahead," Charles said. So we did, and the older women cursed and shook their fists at us. "Haitians believe that being photographed by a *blan* is bad luck," he explained. We passed the collapsed Presidential Palace. More than 20,000 poor Haitians had moved into a camp across the road. There were rows of seeping outhouses, and mountains of toxic waste, pools of stagnant water and ecstatic mosquitos that created a tornado of disease over and around and under everything.

We followed a UN military jeep into a demolished area called Carrefour. A group of children ran after us. "Hey you, hey you," they cried out in English. As we slowed to go around some potholes, they ran to our windows with their hands open, begging for food or money. We wanted to give them something but felt uncertain, not because we thought they were dangerous, but because we did not know the rules of engagement. A group of bigger boys began washing our car windows with rags. Charles turned on the windshield wipers to discourage them, but they ran along the side of the car, imploring us to give them something. A smaller boy washed a window with the torn sleeve of his shirt. "Can we give him a dollar?" someone asked. What we really wanted was to rescue him from this nightmare. He couldn't have been more than 6 years old. The concept of "rescue" would well up over and over in some of us as a conflict in the days and weeks to come. We knew that Haitians did not need rescue; they needed liberation. They did not need white saviors; they needed access to education and opportunities so they could realize their full humanity. But in that moment, confronted with that child, these truths seemed theoretical. This child was real.

We visited the largest camp in Haiti, located on a golf course in an area called Delmas. Over 50,000 people were living there. As we entered the camp a group of children grabbed our hands, dancing and singing "hey you." We stopped every few minutes to speak with anyone willing to talk with us. We learned that even with the huge amount of aid flowing into Haiti, people in the camp were living in terrible conditions. Some had untreated wounds from the quake. Most had no food or clean water. Many said their children were sick, and many children had swollen bellies.

We passed a young mother bathing an infant in a plastic bucket. She told us the baby's father had died in the earthquake and she was alone in the camp. She could not nurse her baby because her milk had "dried up." Her tent was made of rags and sticks. Every time it rained the floor turned to mud and she had to stand all night holding the baby in her arms.

We saw a woman standing alone in the middle of a dirt path. She had the saddest eyes in the world. She told us her house was destroyed, and her husband and two sons had gone to the countryside to live with relatives. Her three daughters were working as maids at the Hotel Montana when it collapsed. "Workers came and dug out the bodies of the blan," she said, "but my daughters are still buried." She told us she would not leave Port au Prince until she could give her daughters a proper burial. We asked Charles if aid workers would dig them out. "No," he said. "Bulldozers will clear them away with the rubble."

Charles said that after the earthquake tens of thousands of dead bodies filled the streets and public squares and fields. The bodies decayed, and the smell of death hung in the air. The government resorted to mass burials in mass graves, using garbage trucks to clear the dead. Vodou priests protested this desecration of the body, this abandonment of sacred tradition in the name of public health. The spirits of the dead will be tormented, they said.

We passed a group of three women balancing tubs of charcoal on their heads and they asked us if we were with an aid organization. We explained we were there to try and understand the situation in Haiti. We could feel their assessment: "What good are you if you have not come with aid?" We asked the oldest how much she earned selling charcoal. On a good day, she might make a dollar. We asked how often she had a meal. "On days we get food we eat," she said. "On days we cannot get food we don't. It's like the proverb says: sometimes things are up and sometimes they are down."

Further along, we met a teenage girl who told us she had been living in the camp with her younger siblings since the quake. Four children hid behind her, emaciated, dirty, and silent. She said their mother had died, and she was the only one who could care for them. She asked us if we could help her. When we told her that we were not from an aid organization, her eyes became hard and she turned her back on us. "I am not in the mood to talk," she told Charles. "I cannot talk anymore. I may not be able to talk tomorrow because there are things that hurt me a lot. I am suffering a lot." We were in Haiti to help, but how? In listening to these testimonies we were bearing witness, but what good was it if we walked away? Of course we could publish a report—*raise awareness*—but how would it help this girl and these lost children?

It was late afternoon when we left the camp. Our next stop was at a public interest law firm in Haiti. The organization had agreed to let us work at their center and camp out in the yard. The director listened carefully as we explained our project to him. We told him that our goal was to understand the human rights situation in Haiti, and to identify people who might qualify for evacuation because of some extraordinary circumstance – displacement alone was not enough. We wanted the most compelling cases, but we did not have time to interview thousands of people to find them. "The key is to outline your priorities," he said. We identified the three most likely categories of cases: people with medical issues that could not be treated in Haiti; orphaned children with biological relatives in the diaspora; elders or disabled individuals with no means of survival in Haiti. The director offered to connect our team with a coalition of women's organizations working in camps in Port au Prince.

We met with three Haitian women leaders. They confirmed on a large scale what we had witnessed that day. Many Haitians were malnourished, but food distribution had stopped. There were serious medical, security, and sanitation problems in the camps, which they described as lawless and violent. Given our impression that the world had pledged billions in aid to help Haiti, we couldn't understand why there was no food or security. "There is a lack of communication between the government, the United Nations and NGOs," they said. We asked if they had attended any of the UN coordination meetings we'd heard about. "The blan conduct the meetings in French," they explained. "We speak Creole."

Working

Our first night in Haiti we slept in tents within the compound where we would be working. The women leaders arrived at seven the next morning with around 30 of their "most serious cases." There were mothers with children, children with grandparents, siblings without parents, two amputees, and a group of adolescent girls. We learned that the families were from areas called Martissant, Bel Aire, Cite Soleil, and Gran Ravine. In these areas, 95 % of people lived on less than a dollar a day. Most children did not go to school. Most adults did not know how to read or write. Everyone was struggling with daily survival. Everyone was grieving.

We interviewed five women, all widows who had lost their husbands in the quake. Sanitation workers had loaded their bodies into dump trucks and taken them to a mass grave. Two of the women had also lost children, one had lost her parents, and one had lost her sister. We interviewed four teenagers, all orphans who had lost parents in the disaster. Two had lost their whole families, one had lost four sisters, and one asked if we could help find her sister. "She started talking nonsense after our mother died," she said. "She started walking around naked and she walked off and is missing." We interviewed an elder who told us her daughters had died and she was taking care of her grandchildren. The toddlers had swollen bellies and infected eyes.

Most of the women and children had undiagnosed psychiatric symptoms. One woman said there were black wings beating inside her head and black spots before her eyes. Another felt a constant rumble in her ears, "like a train, or something breaking apart in there." Another had been gasping for breath ever since being trapped under rubble. One had a racing heartbeat; another itched from head to toe. A mother reported that her daughter talked to walls and heard voices that were not there. A teenage orphan said he had unrelenting stomach cramps. An old woman said her sister had a droop to the left side of her face and had "walked at a tilt ever since the earthquake." A young girl said, "Sometimes it feels like my head is being detached from my body, and it makes me want to run away." We asked her how often that happened and she said, "Whenever I think of the dead bodies."

By the end of the morning we had screened over a dozen people and two dozen more had arrived. The sun bore down on the people sitting on folding chairs, but no one complained. We established a three-step process. First, an interpreter gathered basic biographical information from each person. Then, a lawyer obtained a complete psychosocial history covering three periods—pre-quake, during the quake, and post-quake. If the case presented an extraordinary circumstance—medical, psychological, or psychosocial—the lawyers referred the case to the psychiatrists.

Almost all of the cases presented extraordinary circumstances. Many people had tragic stories from before the earthquake. We interviewed one woman who said members of the FRAPH—a paramilitary group that opposed Jean-Bertrand Aristide—had killed her husband and raped her and her three daughters because they had supported Aristide. We interviewed another woman who was shot in the leg. The FRAPH murdered her husband. Another woman said that she had lost three husbands: members of the paramilitary killed the first, the second drowned while trying to escape Haiti on a sloop, and the third died in the quake.

We met a woman named Rose. She wore a blue-flowered dress that hung like a sack over her bony shoulders. Her muscles were wasted from malnutrition. She wore leather sandals, and her feet were caked with dirt. One of her ankles was swollen the size of a melon, and she winced in pain when she walked. We learned that four teenage boys had raped her 2 days after the earthquake. She was 58 years old. She had been trying to rescue a young girl they were attacking, and the boys had turned on her and gang-raped her. They had crushed her ankle during the rape. She had not received medical care. She sat stooped over in her chair as she reported this history through an interpreter. "I am carrying bleach in my purse," she said in a low voice. "Tomorrow maybe I will drink it." Tears filled her eyes as she raised her face, seeking some sign of hope that would be stronger than her wish to die.

Rose was not the only shattered one. We interviewed a woman named Claire who said her husband had died in the earthquake and she was caring for two children, a boy who had been mute since witnessing a massacre in 2004 and a girl who had stopped speaking after the earthquake. Claire told us she was raped in the Champs de Mars camp and was pregnant. She was still sleeping in the camp where she was attacked, which added another dimension to her trauma.

By the end of our first day we had evaluated more than two dozen cases. We worked with the Haitian women leaders to coordinate whatever psychosocial support we could cobble together. Two of our interpreters offered to allow four teenage orphans caring for babies to stay with them. One woman leader took Rose home with her. Another looked after Claire. These women had survived this way for generations—Haitians helping Haitians. We understood our role was to support these leaders, not replace them. If we wanted to help Haiti, we needed to work through local community-based organizations that could guide us in our efforts.

> *"We understood our role was to support these leaders, not replace them. If we wanted to help Haiti, we needed to work through local community-based organizations that could guide us in our efforts."*

Dark and Deeper Dark

On our second full day of work, all of the folding chairs in the courtyard were filled by half past six in the morning. There were many people, and they kept coming. We interviewed a woman named Claudette who told us that she was 50 years old and from Cite Soleil. The FRAPH had murdered her husband, raped her, and shot her daughter. Her son died in the earthquake, and her home was destroyed. Claudette and her daughters moved to a camp on a soccer field, but "bandits" set fire to the camp and threatened to kill anyone who returned there. She moved to a yard in an area called Little Haiti, but bandits there were raping and killing people. Claudette tried to help several rape victims by taking them to the hospital. Later bandits threatened her with death for doing this. One day her cousin was selling cold drinks on the street, and a man walked up and shot her in the chest. Neighbors took her to St. Catherine's Hospital in a pushcart, but she did not survive. People in the area made a police report, but they did not investigate. Claudette thought the man shot her cousin because she had helped a rape victim. Now she had no place to go. "My friends used to tell me to have faith," she said. "Now they say I would be better off dead."

We learned that "bandits" were raping women and girls in the most dangerous areas every night. We interviewed a 17-year-old girl, Joanne, who had lost her parents and grandparents and cousins in the earthquake. Her sister was missing. Joanne told us she was walking in the street crying, and a man stopped her and asked her what was wrong. She told him her story, and he said that his sister could take care of her. She was convinced that God had sent the man to her, so she went with him to his house. There was no sister. Three men raped her. "They did not kill me, but I am dead inside," she said.

We met a woman named Yolande who described how she was raped and then her two daughters were raped after the earthquake. "I thought about killing myself and my children," she said. "I thought about buying a gallon of bleach and using it as water. I would drink a cup and give the children a cup. Once I bought bleach and I was making spaghetti and I put bleach in the spaghetti." The children refused to eat the spaghetti. But there were other dangers. "Sometimes I do actions that I don't have any control over," Yolande said. "The other day my daughter made me mad. I threw a knife at her and she was bleeding. I don't know how I could have done that."

It was hard to listen to such narratives. We wanted to help but often felt powerless. The psychiatrists could diagnose psychiatric and medical conditions and write evaluations, but they could not provide treatment. The lawyers could prepare humanitarian parole cases based on the med/psych evaluations, but there was no guarantee the US government would grant them. We tried to help patients obtain access to care in Haiti, but capacity was severely limited or unavailable.

The work was especially hard on our five Haitian interpreters. One night the psychiatrists held an impromptu debriefing session with them to assess how they were handling the intensity of the interviews. Although all of them had worked as fixers for the foreign press, none of them had worked in mental health or with victims of persecution and rape or in a post-disaster setting. They had all suffered losses in the earthquake, and hearing story after story of death and suffering was inevitably re-traumatizing. Four of the interpreters were eager to open up to the psychiatrists and learn coping skills. Charles slipped away when the exchange turned personal. "I'm not the type to talk about my feelings," he said later. As tough as he was, we worried about him. He was sleeping in his car. He told us he did not have any family. He had complained of a migraine earlier that day. We suspected he needed more than aspirin.

Medical

One morning we went to the General Hospital with Charles to try and obtain basic medical care for four rape victims we had interviewed the day before. When we pulled up, a group of amputees were begging on the road outside the hospital compound. Inside, a crowd of mothers and children waited to be seen in tents that served as pediatric examining rooms. Some children surrounded us as we passed, begging for food and money. We asked a guard for directions to the area for gynecology, and he pointed to a part of the hospital that had not collapsed. We entered a large room with long corridors leading off in different directions. Dozens of patients were sitting on the floor, lying in the corridors, sitting under blown-out windows. Some ignored us. Some stared at us with hard eyes. A Haitian nurse was hustling about. We asked her where we should sign in. She waved us to a station down the hall. We passed several empty examining rooms, but there was no sign of a doctor. A receptionist took the names of our patients and told us to wait. We waited. The place was dark and dirty and smelled of urine. Every now and then a clerk appeared and tossed medical records into broken cardboard boxes lined up against the wall. An hour passed and no doctor appeared. More patients arrived, and we waited. After 2 hours we asked the receptionist when the doctor would come. "He might come today," she said. "He might come?" we asked. Charles said something to her in Creole and she shrugged her shoulders. "He might come," Charles repeated. We ushered our four patients back to the car.

By now it was midday. We drove to a private clinic, but they told us they did not handle rape cases. We drove to a clinic run by Medecines Sans Frontieres (MSF) near the Champs de Mars camp, but their team had left for the day. The coordinator there sent us to another MSF clinic across town. Dozens of patients were lined up outside the fenced tent clinic. Some were alone and others had helpers; some children were carried, some cried, some were mute. We thought about what to do. It was late in the day. It was critical for the girls to get prophylactic care within 72 hours of the rapes. Hundreds of eyes followed us as we walked to the front of the line where a Haitian guard controlled admission. Charles explained that we were Americans bringing patients who needed urgent care. The guard unbolted the gate, let us in, and slammed it behind us. We did not have the courage to look into the eyes of the desperate Haitian mothers locked outside, holding sick children in their arms.

It's important to cultivate detachment when you do this work, bearing witness to such terrible suffering. It's important to allow another person's suffering to pass through you, rather than become trapped in you, so that you are not too overwhelmed to help in practical ways. Detachment was impossible for some of us in Haiti. The worst thing was that the need for help was overwhelming and our capacity to make a difference was small. We knew that we would have to focus our project in a way that would allow us to leverage resources—academic and professional—and employ our specialized skills to the greatest possible advantage. We left Haiti the next day with this goal in our mind.

Focus

During our first week in Haiti we interviewed 124 people. We identified 37 candidates for humanitarian parole. What is important about our first delegation is that we documented patterns of harm that would guide us in our advocacy. As in many humanitarian disasters, women and children were the most vulnerable populations. As in many countries, gender-based violence was one of the greatest threats to them. All 37 candidates we agreed to help were rape victims. Many were raped multiple times and had family members who were raped. All had a clear diagnosis of post-traumatic stress disorder (PTSD), and some were suicidal. We decided to help this subgroup because we considered them the most likely to become victims of repeat violence or harm. Their defenses were reduced to nothing; their access to protection was non-existent.

By focusing on gender-based violence cases, we also hoped to utilize our areas of professional expertise to bridge a gap not filled by mega-NGOs working on the emergency relief effort. We aimed to offer support to local, grassroots women's groups that were sometimes overlooked by large foreign aid organizations. We were committed to a bottom-up approach that would empower rather than disable local leaders who had been engaged in a decades-long fight to protect Haitian women and girls.

Returning

The predominant emotion after our first delegation to Haiti was a longing to go back. Part of this was motivated by a desire to strengthen our relationships with leaders on the ground, an indispensable element of any project. Part was motivated by a desire to return to the women we had identified for humanitarian parole and do more detailed interviews for their legal cases. Besides these reasons, we felt compelled to return because our work felt purposeful. Perhaps when you witness such enormous suffering that is the most you can do – work with purpose. And so we did.

We returned to Haiti four times in 2010. Our list of humanitarian parole candidates swelled to over 50. Several hundred women and girls were raped in camps that year. The youngest victim we interviewed was 5 years old. The oldest was 65. We documented a growing phenomenon of girls selling their bodies for food or shelter. When they became pregnant some of them ingested bleach or poisonous herbs to try to abort the babies. Many ended up in hospital emergency rooms, and some died. In the first 6 months of our project, three of our clients died—two from lack of access to medical care and one from refusing medical treatment after a rape.

In the beginning, our team consisted of both psychiatrists and lawyers on the ground. This enabled us to identify life-threatening medical issues, extreme mental health pathologies, and suicide risks. Later, when doctors were not available to travel to Haiti with us, we devised a system that enabled teams in Haiti to communicate with them remotely. Every time we took a new legal case, psychiatrists from Stanford conducted a psychological evaluation by Skype. This served several purposes: it allowed the lawyers to triage legal cases on the basis of severity of diagnosis, develop forensic evidence for legal submissions, and corroborate the testimonies of our clients.

The psychiatrists conducted not only evaluations at the beginning of a case but also follow-up evaluations on clients waiting for their cases to be adjudicated. Part of this was so that the lawyers did not have to submit "stale" evaluations with cases. Part was to show that the clients still needed mental health care that was not available in Haiti. Many were living in safe houses for which the project paid, so they were out of the immediate danger of camps. Still, their PTSD had not healed itself. While this may seem obvious to clinicians, it was not at all obvious to legal adjudicators. The evaluations became important supplemental evidence.

One afternoon we arranged for psychiatry to re-evaluate Rose, the older woman who was gang-raped after the quake. A year had passed since her first evaluation and she was living in one of our safe houses. She was wearing a beautiful African tunic and matching headdress. She was no longer stooped over or unclean. Her ankle was healing. She peered into the screen of the laptop, squinting at the fuzzy image of the doctors conducting the evaluation. They greeted her warmly and asked how she was feeling. She gave them the sweetest smile in the world and said, "I'm not carrying bleach in my purse anymore." She was like a child and an old woman and an angel all wrapped into one.

Despite her renewed hope, the outcomes of the evaluations were troubling. The women the psychiatrists interviewed over Skype had crossed the bridge from acute to chronic PTSD. Although they had more coping skills, they still suffered flashbacks, sleeplessness, nightmares, and panic attacks. They still lacked the ability to concentrate, were easily startled, and were pulled back into the black vortex of pain whenever they felt threatened. One woman said, "Whenever I hear about a rape it is like I am being raped all over again." We asked how often this happened. "Every day," she said.

Psychological evaluations like this one, coupled with legal arguments for humanitarian protection, gave our project enormous credibility. It was time to engage in broader advocacy.

Advocacy

In the summer of 2010, we met with the leaders of the United Nations High Commissioner for Refugees (UNHCR) in Washington, DC to relay what we had witnessed in Haiti. We described the terrifying situation in the camps. Little children were being raped. Orphans were selling their bodies for food. Young woman were being kidnapped and mutilated. Community leaders attempting to protect victims faced constant death threats and retaliatory violence. We referred to the structural failures that contributed to the problem. There were no government-run shelters for rape victims. Free medical care was nonexistent. The police were indifferent to sexual violence, shamed victims, and refused to investigate crimes without a bribe.

The prosecution rate for rape was under 2 %. This climate of impunity fueled the crisis, where criminals knew that if they raped a woman or a girl or a child there would be no penalty. We did not have a specific "ask" during that meeting, but urged UNHCR to address the lack of protection for women and girls. They said they were aware of the crisis and working on a protection plan.

The next month, we met with the UNHCR team in Haiti to continue the advocacy started in Washington. We were just finishing another week in Port au Prince and wanted to provide information about what we'd seen. The meeting was at first awkward and formal. They were experts; we were strangers in a foreign land. We talked about our clients who had been kidnapped or raped or become pregnant from rapes. We described women carrying bleach in their purse, clients who had died, and girls selling their bodies for food. We explained that we'd interviewed hundreds of women and children since the earthquake and carefully documented their stories.

As the meeting progressed, the tone shifted. The UNHCR team talked of the limits of their mission and the need for more accurate data. They spoke of the debate that existed around rape in Haiti, with some claiming that victims were making false reports to obtain resources, and others claiming that the problem was dramatically underreported. It was impossible to know where to draw the line. Some studies were empirically flawed. Some media reports were sensationalized and inaccurate. They asked what areas of the city we were working in and what patterns we were seeing in which areas. They asked what methods we used to test the credibility of cases and how we gathered forensic evidence.

We explained that we conducted multiple interviews with every client and that Stanford psychiatrists conducted psychological evaluations in every case. We knew that clients sometimes embellished stories to obtain benefits, but we had forensic medical evidence in our cases and did not believe any of our clients had fabricated stories. At the end of our meeting, the UNHCR team said they would welcome further discussion and suggested we meet the next time we were in town.

Over the next year, we met with UNHCR every chance we had, both in Port au Prince and Washington. We described what we were witnessing in the camps and pleaded with them to support our cases. We learned they were talking to people in the US State Department about a possible resettlement program for Haitians. They were also talking with the Canadian government. The focus of the talks centered on cases involving gender-based violence after the earthquake. These classified talks gave us hope.

Resettlement

In 2011, we filed our first four humanitarian parole cases with the US Department of Homeland Security (DHS). All of the cases involved rapes, kidnappings, and murders. One of the cases involved multiple generations of rapes and the murder of four family members. Three of the cases involved pregnancies from rapes. We had lined up host families and organizations willing to support all of the clients.

Stanford provided support in the form of psychiatric evaluation for every case. But that was not all. Simultaneously with our filings, UNHCR agreed to submit letters of support to DHS, urging it to allow our families to come to the states. A month later, we had our first victory. By the end of the year, we had won all four cases. The families were evacuated in late 2011.

In January 2012, we were back in Haiti. In the 2 years since the earthquake, our teams had traveled there nearly a dozen times. We continued to gather evidence for our legal cases. Although we had evacuated four of our most at-risk families, we had over 50 more in grave crisis. Some clients were angry because they had not been evacuated yet, although we never made any promises. Some tried to convince us that they should be evacuated next because their cases were the most serious. Some prayed to their Gods that they would be the next ones to leave. We had not been able to identify hosts for these clients, so we could not even file their humanitarian parole cases, much less prioritize who was first. We were paying for food and safe houses for all of the clients, but this depended upon the charity of friends and colleagues. "Disasters have a one year shelf life," a friend had said. The year was up. We were paying Charles to watch over the clients in our absence. He did everything from managing safe houses to obtaining identity documents to registering children in primary school. We had hired the head of a local women's group to take clients for medical care and hired another woman to support our young mothers with new-borns. We could not have sustained the project without these community-based leaders. They kept our clients alive while we built cases and waited for legal decisions. We did everything we could to keep people stable, but we were treading water. We were constantly worried that if we ran out of money our clients would fall back into a life of extreme poverty and violence and despair.

Loss

Two years after the earthquake, we were back on the ground in Haiti. By now, a dozen or so lawyers had gone with us to interview victims and gather evidence. One day we were meeting with clients and a taxi driver showed up with two young men and an older woman. The woman was stretched out in the back of the driver's pickup truck moaning. The men were holding her hands and comforting her. "Help her," one pleaded. "What happened?" we asked. The men told us that the woman was their mother and she had been gang-raped after trying to rescue their sister from an attack. She was so badly hurt that she could not walk. The attack had happened the night before. They brought her to us because they had heard that our project would pay for medical care. We paid the taxi driver, took basic biographical information, and sent the woman to the hospital with our medical liaison. We paid for X-rays and blood transfusions. The men stayed at their mother's side for 2 days and nights. She died on the third day.

We met with UNHCR in Port au Prince again that week. We told them the situation was getting worse. Charles interpreted in French. He rarely offered his own opinions in these meetings, but that day he was visibly shaken and angry.

He completed sentences we were too diplomatic to complete. He described the suffering of the clients and demanded to know what the United Nations was going to do about it. He was the only Haitian in the room. No one dared to question him.

The next week we got a call from UNHCR in DC. "Send us some cases," they said. "We may have a deal with Canada." They said that 50 families would be selected for resettlement in Montreal. Fifteen spaces were reserved for our project. Thirteen of our families were selected for evacuation. Two cases we referred did not meet the criteria: candidates had to be internally displaced persons (IDPs) who had suffered gender-based violence after the earthquake. The two rejected cases involved murders and rapes from before the disaster. Although these clients were at least as traumatized as the others, they were on the wrong side of the line in the sand. We asked if we could submit alternative cases to reach the threshold of 15 (we had dozens more) but were told it was too late. Those slots had been given to other projects.

Endings

Months turned into years in Haiti, and we could never find a path to the exit. During the first 3 years of the project, we evacuated more clients and raised more money to protect the ones left behind in Haiti. We wrote heartfelt reflections and shared them with friends and donors. We told stories about girls being kidnapped and gang-raped. We recalled a mother who had given her baby away to a foreigner because she could not feed her. We asked rhetorical questions about our humanitarian duty to protect the most vulnerable ones. We dismissed the notion that Haiti was a basket case and urged people to help. We shared accounts of how Haitian women were banding together to protect one another, despite huge risks of retaliatory violence. By the fourth year of the project, we were out of words. We were also out of money. Although UNHCR and several friends and colleagues had provided funding for our safe houses in 2012–2013, those grants had ended. The Canada project was coming to a close. Our local project leaders were exhausted.

In early 2014, we talked about whether it was time to conclude our project. We had responded to the disaster in Haiti the best we could. We had permanently resettled 60 women and children in the United

> "We had developed a model that could be transferred to any humanitarian crisis in the world."

States and Canada. We had developed a model that could be transferred to any humanitarian crisis in the world. This is the structure: a partnership between psychiatrists, lawyers, community-based leaders, and UNHCR aimed at providing a holistic response to humanitarian crisis. At its core, it is a kind of global refugee clinic that travels to the victim of persecution rather than waiting for the victim to escape across a border or an ocean or a continent to seek protection. With telehealth technology now globally accessible, academic psychiatrists can be effective in this model without travel, thus maximizing their capacity. Our team looks next to other global situations to explore the utility of our blueprint for humanitarian parole for survivors of gender based violence.

With more than 50 million refugees in the world today and untold numbers of survivors of gender-based violence, the concept may seem an inconsequential remedy. To Yolande and Claire and Joanne and the 50 other women and children evacuated to the United States and Canada, it was the difference between life and death.

Narrative 15
Voices of Experience

Laura Weiss Roberts

We asked academic faculty colleagues who work closely with community partners to comment on aspects of their collaborations. We explored how partnerships are important and how to best approach partnerships. We asked about the strengths and barriers in collaboration. We also inquired about what academic faculty colleagues wished they had known at the beginning of their collaborative work. What follows are some "pearls of wisdom" from their lived experiences in partnerships.

Question: Can You Say a Bit About Why Community-Academic Partnerships Are Important to You and to Your Work?

Community-academic partnerships can address questions that uniquely impact community members. Each partner brings specific expertise and skills that are necessary in developing approaches and interventions to solve complicated biomedical and psychosocial problems in a manner that is culturally appropriate and sensitive.

Cheryl Gore-Felton, Ph.D.

Contributing authors: Steven Adelsheim, M.D., Michele Barry, M.D., Victor G. Carrion, M.D., Jack Drescher, M.D., Cheryl Gore-Felton, Ph.D., Keith Humphreys, Ph.D., Shashank V. Joshi, M.D., Cheryl Koopman, Ph.D., Joseph B. Layde, M.D., J.D., Yvonne Aida Maldonado, M.D., Lawrence McGlynn, M.S., M.D., Daryn Reicherter, M.D., and David Wyatt Seal, Ph.D.

L.W. Roberts, M.D. M.A. (✉)
Department of Psychiatry and Behavioral Sciences, Stanford University School of Medicine, Stanford, CA, USA
e-mail: RobertsL@stanford.edu

© Springer International Publishing Switzerland 2015
L.W. Roberts et al. (eds.), *Partnerships for Mental Health*,
DOI 10.1007/978-3-319-18884-3_15

As those in academia learn from and respect the intrinsic knowledge, voice, and experience of those in the community, the strengths of all are brought together to create elegant solutions.

Steven Adelsheim, M.D.

Community-academic partnerships ground academicians to the real world and open the community to the struggles of research.

Michele Barry, M.D.

In order for academic work (e.g., research, program development) to create impact, the work needs to be significant, feasible, and sustainable. Community-academic partnerships engage stakeholders in this process. This relationship safeguards that these components are addressed during design, implementation, and evaluation of an intervention or program.

Victor G. Carrion, M.D.

Growing up in a Christian church, I was taught that "faith without works is dead." In my university career, I have learned that "scholarship without service is dead." Mental health is not physics: We are rarely discovering how an electron works or some other bit of basic knowledge. Instead, we strive to acquire knowledge in the service of society. That by definition means engaging society at all levels.

Keith Humphreys, Ph.D.

Research and academic training that are not rooted in community needs, values, and priorities are doomed to failure. Transcendent collaborations that uniquely synthesize scientific and programmatic expertise increase the likelihood of developing an intervention or program that is scientifically efficacious, programmatically valid, and responsive to community needs, values, and priorities.

David Wyatt Seal, Ph.D.

It is important to me because the university setting is often full of researchers and clinicians who want to help the community and who may have burning questions for which the community may have some answers (and more questions). Hence, a dialogue can start, and a mutually beneficial relationship can be created and sustained. Also, I think it's particularly salient when you live in the community where you work…you become part of the landscape and the research questions become more natural and obvious.

Shashank V. Joshi, M.D.

Academic endeavors must ultimately provide some benefit, whether direct or indirect, to the general population and, sometimes, to specific communities. Partnering with these communities will enrich the nature of the academic inquiry and lead to more robust applications.

Yvonne Aida Maldonado, M.D.

I have had a rewarding, synergistic experience between my professional work—in which I try to serve my profession in its desire to provide greater understanding and better treatment of the mental health needs of LGBT patients—while serving my gay community as an occasional spokesperson to the wider world in support of their civil rights, health, and mental health needs.

Jack Drescher, M.D.

As a vice chairman for education and director of a forensic psychiatry fellowship, I tremendously value the ability to expose learners at all stages of medical education to patients and clinical problems in the real world. Community engagement with the corrections system, public hospitals, the Veterans Affairs medical center system, and universities where student mental health services are provided all give opportunities to medical students, residents, and fellows to prepare for careers serving patients in the environments where they receive care in the community.

Joseph B. Layde, M.D., J.D.

The connection between methamphetamine use disorders and HIV/AIDS has been well documented in the literature. Scientists at major academic centers have utilized fMRI, brain tissue analysis from autopsies, neuropsychological testing, and a variety of other scientific approaches to understand addiction and the effects of methamphetamine in those with and without HIV/AIDS. Communities, however, see methamphetamine causing friends and loved ones to participate in unsafe sex, commit crime, become homeless, and in some cases, develop recurring psychosis and debilitating depression.

I see the marriage of academia and community as a critical link between the abstract and the concrete. This union provides a venue where fMRI results are understood in the context of community observations, such as why a college student would decide not to use a condom when under the influence of methamphetamine. The observations of the local bathhouse employee are given as much cachet as a research scientist. The community learns from academia and vice versa.

Lawrence McGlynn, M.D.

Community-academic partnerships provide community leaders with an approach to help shape research that addresses their community's needs. Community-academic partnerships can facilitate the implementation of research by drawing upon the community partners' extensive knowledge of their community and building upon their already well-established relationships within it.

Cheryl Koopman, Ph.D.

I am dedicated to forging community-academic partnerships. Without these relationships I could not create the synergy needed to best serve the community populations I work with. I have worked on both sides of the relationship, and now my charge is to wear both hats simultaneously. The synergy I can achieve is unbelievable. But the balance is sometimes a challenge. And acting as liaison twixt the two can be fun and often humorous. Sometimes each partner has such a different mind-set, it's as though they are from different planets but have the same ultimate goal. I sometimes feel like a translator or, better yet, an ambassador.

Daryn Reicherter, M.D.

Questions: How Does Someone Learn to Engage with Communities in a Manner That Is Respectful and Leads to Strong Partnerships? How Did You Learn?

By being curious and learning about their mission and their process. By being hum-ble and recognizing that one may not have anything to contribute to an existing system, but one may most definitely have something to learn.

Victor G. Carrion, M.D.

My approach to engaging communities in my academic endeavors is to identify a key leader in the community who is trusted and respected and to work with that person to build a bilateral relationship. By that I mean that, while the research out-comes might not always directly and immediately impact the community, there would be some type of indirect benefit to the community, such as skills building, mentorship, or other opportunities.

Yvonne Aida Maldonado, M.D.

The best way to learn how to work with a community in a respectful manner is to work with someone who is doing it well. This is how I learned.

Cheryl Gore-Felton, Ph.D.

First, find the "elder" of the community and engage in dialogue. Second, listen to their needs and not yours. Third, you never can become culturally competent but one can learn cultural humility.

Michele Barry, M.D.

Understand what the community's needs are from their vantage point. Ask the com-munity members for their ideas on how to approach the issues. Don't be afraid to ask the members what certain terms mean, but speaking their vernacular may be seen as patronizing. Do not be apologetic for our academic standing—in the academic-community partnership, members usually take pride in the accomplish-ments of other members.

As in many areas of life, I learned my lessons by trial and error. I also attended a number of national conferences, leading to working relationships with subject-matter experts, and I continue to benefit from their expertise. Much of my learning, however, came from my own mistakes. At one point I lost a significant number of group members. I could not understand why, for I had made their lives easier by doing much of the grunt work myself. As a result of my actions, they felt left out and obsolete. Luckily, the community is a forgiving lot, and they did not stay away for too long.

Lawrence McGlynn, M.D.

Academic psychiatry and community psychiatry have to be approached with the same level of respect. Whether these groups are formally collaborating or not, they are partners in mental health. We are all colleagues. We should sit at a round table without hierarchy. I learned this by doing it for my whole academic and community career.

Daryn Reicherter, M.D.

I draw upon resources from the literature (such as [1]) that suggest several elements to the participatory partnership:

- Recognizes community as a unit of identity
- Builds upon strengths and resources within the community
- Facilitates collaborative partnership in all phases of the research
- Integrates knowledge and action for mutual benefit of all partners
- Promotes a co-learning and empowering process that attends to social inequalities
- Involves a cyclic and iterative process
- Addresses health from both positive and ecological perspectives
- Disseminates findings gained to all partners

David Wyatt Seal, Ph.D.

A major source of learning how to engage with a community partner is to pay attention to what the community partner says and does. Key actions for showing respect are active listening and expressing appreciation for actions taken on behalf of the project. Keeping promises builds trust and strengthens partnerships.

The funding agency for much of my community-based research …does an outstanding job of educating both academic and community partners in how to build strong partnerships. This education has been provided through conference and workshop presentations, newsletters and other educational materials, and conference calls in which the program officer checks in with community and academic partners. I have also learned a great deal about how to engage with my community partners from reading what others have published on related topics such as on community-based participatory research.

Cheryl Koopman, Ph.D.

Willingness to be taught and acknowledgement of one's own ignorance are prerequisites for learning. Universities do not always nurture these traits in faculty, so one must unlearn the socialization we are subject to as "academic experts" and admit that there are many things we don't know and there are many people who know them but don't have fancy letters after their name. Professors are supposed to profess, but I have personally learned more in my community work when I talked less and listened more.

Keith Humphreys, Ph.D.

Question: What Are Some of the Things That You Have Observed That Get in the Way of Partnership-Building?

Although integration of systems is good in concept, the idea may be threatening to the identity of existing organizations, especially if these identities have been built to hold a certain amount of power and personal capital. Cooperation, co-location, and collaboration are more tolerable terms and may organically lead to integration.

Victor G. Carrion, M.D.

Mistrust. Often I have gone into communities where I was not the first researcher to come, and there were hard feelings left over from previous experiences. In these instances, I had to learn patience and to build my relationships with key community members over time. Finances and resources can also get in the way of building effective partnerships. It is important to treat community partners as key personnel on the project with salary support, resources, and positions that demonstrate a true partnership. The manner in which the data are analyzed and interpreted can break the strongest of relationships if not discussed early in the partnership development and throughout the project. Community interests may not line up with research or scientific interests, and balancing these perspectives is important.

Cheryl Gore-Felton, Ph.D.

Arrogance. Ideology. Rigidity. Political tone deafness. Grandiosity. Self-righteousness. Inability or unwillingness to say, "I don't know" or "I'm truly sorry." They are all unhelpful, on either side of the academic/community divide.

Jack Drescher, M.D.

Poor communication around goal sets and expectations can cause rifts. My experience is that the academic's goals should always be in keeping with the mission of the partner. For instance, if an academic wants to develop a training opportunity for residents and the community partner wants clinical time, this could be a "win-win" for both groups. But poor communication could misconstrue the process. Also being clear in communication about data collection is important. This also should be a "win-win" for both groups, yet, if poorly communicated, this can lead to the impression that the relationship is one-sided (the academic center grabbing data and leaving).

Daryn Reicherter, M.D.

There are, at times, different agendas held by community partners and educational institutions. Understandably, community organizations hope to obtain excellent medical services through affiliation with a medical school, whereas they may not be as tuned into the realities of medical education in the medical school setting. Working through those issues of sometimes competing agendas is important and, if not done correctly, can get in the way of partnership building.

Joseph B. Layde, M.D., J.D.

In the end, I think turf, ownership, control, and ego are the main partners. Most "community-academic partnerships" involve doing *to* or doing *for*, not doing *with*. Transcendent partnership involves community working *with* academia toward common shared goals. Issues to address and resolve include ownership and control; research versus service delivery; time orientation; ensuring program/research integrity; overcoming status quo; gaining broad-based support; overreliance on being experts; funding versus community priorities; and competition for existing community resources.

David Wyatt Seal, Ph.D.

Question: What Are the Three Things You Wish You Had Known When You First Started Doing Work With Communities?

I wish I would have known to be patient. Like any important relationship, it takes time to build a trusting and collaborative relationship with community partners. One meeting may not be enough. In fact, you might have to attend some community events, even those that at the time do not seem relevant to your interests.

Find the gatekeeper. Every community has a person who is the social glue. It is the person who knows the key people in the community who are the decision makers or who influence the decision makers. Once you find the gatekeeper, recruit them to be part of the team. Their presence on the project helps to build trust with community members, enabling the community to feel comfortable with the research team.

Create partnerships across all aspects of the project. This includes the planning phase and, in some instances, the grant writing phase. Ideally, community members should have key roles on the project and share in the resources and finances of the project. An example of this is when I test a novel intervention in the community, I will hire a community member to be an interventionist. Usually, this person is part of a venue (e.g., clinic, community center, community-based organization) where the study is taking place. This enables the knowledge to remain in the community and assists in the uptake and dissemination of effective interventions. It also reduces the perception that researchers just want to "take" from the community to "build their own careers" and give nothing back. Indeed, there is often a sense that research can partner with a community in ways that enhance quality of life and improve health outcomes.

Cheryl Gore-Felton, M.D.

First, I wish I had known that in many community settings (e.g., schools, public housing projects, social service agencies) people have already had the experience of being studied before and not getting anything out of it. One thus often has to over-come the understandable belief among some community members that research will not be of value to them.

Second, I wish I had known how useless many theories developed in the rarified atmosphere of academia are in communities and therefore that dropping these conceptual frameworks was sometimes necessary to truly understand what was going on.

Third, I underestimated the amount of knowledge already present in communities and took a while to realize that I had as much or more to learn from them as I did to teach.

Keith Humphreys, Ph.D.

How to speak every language in the world.

How the money structure in public health works and the nature of the competition for limited mental health dollars, private and public.

That patience and a yielding attitude are more valuable than any other asset. Lao Tzu asks, "Do you have the patience to wait till your mud settles and the water is clear? Can you remain unmoving till the right action arises by itself?" He must have had these partnerships in mind!

Daryn Reicherter, M.D.

Question: How Has Working with Communities Changed the Nature or Effect of Your Work?

Bringing health care access and equitable care to different cultural communities has been the core of my career.

Michele Barry, M.D.

I have been able to examine complex psychological and social problems in ways that would not have been possible without my community partners. I would not have been able to develop an adolescent HIV prevention intervention for teens living in low-income housing developments or work with men and women living with HIV/AIDS and experiencing trauma symptoms. The community organizations and the people who devote their time to the mission of service have enabled me to create interventions that directly impact the lives of the people who participate. I have adopted and have been adopted by several communities where I have worked. This type of personal connection makes the work very meaningful. It is no longer just about the results of study, but it is about the lives of the participants and the communities in which they live. Many partnerships translate into long-lasting friendships that extend beyond the last participant and the last paper written.

Cheryl Gore-Felton, Ph.D.

Early in one's career, it usually feels inherently good to succeed by academic criteria (e.g., your latest paper comes out). But as time goes by, most people ask themselves "Who cares?" For me, the answer to that is in the community and not in the university. Even though I am proud, for example, of the research I have done on community-based self-help groups for chronic diseases, my greatest sense of "meaning" comes from my direct contact with the people in those groups, seeing them better manage their illness, forge happier lives, and take care of each other.

Keith Humphreys, Ph.D.

For those in academic environments, a successful community partnership brings personal satisfaction unlike those found in any other academic endeavor. Community partnerships keep those of us in academia grounded in the core values and intentions that often led us to our careers.

Steven Adelsheim, M.D.

It is the cornerstone for effectiveness in both my academic capacity and in my ability to create change in public mental health.

Daryn Reicherter, M.D.

Dealing with the fiscal realities of community organizations has made me sensitive to how psychiatric care can take place outside of the academic ivory tower. For instance, learning about different limitations on the pharmacological formularies of prisons, county hospitals, and VA medical centers has made me more sensitive to real-world limitations on the possibilities of affordable care. I think it is also important for medical trainees to be exposed to those realities.

Joseph B. Layde, M.D., J.D.

My work has always been about community partnership. However, I think I have gained significant appreciation for what it takes to develop and build transcendent partnership being in academia.

David Wyatt Seal, Ph.D.

Reference

1. Israel BA, Schulz AJ, Parker EA, Becker AB. Review of community-based research: assessing partnership approaches to improve public health. Annu Rev Public Health. 1998;19:173–202.

Index

© Springer International Publishing Switzerland 2015
L.W. Roberts et al. (eds.), *Partnerships for Mental Health*,
DOI 10.1007/978-3-319-18884-3